ULTIMATE DIABETIC DIET AFTER 50

Finally Live a Healthy Lifestyle With Over 100 Tasty and Healthy Recipes With a Low Glycemic Index. 28 Days Meal Plan.

Emil Gunner

TABLE OF CONTENTS

INTRODUCTION

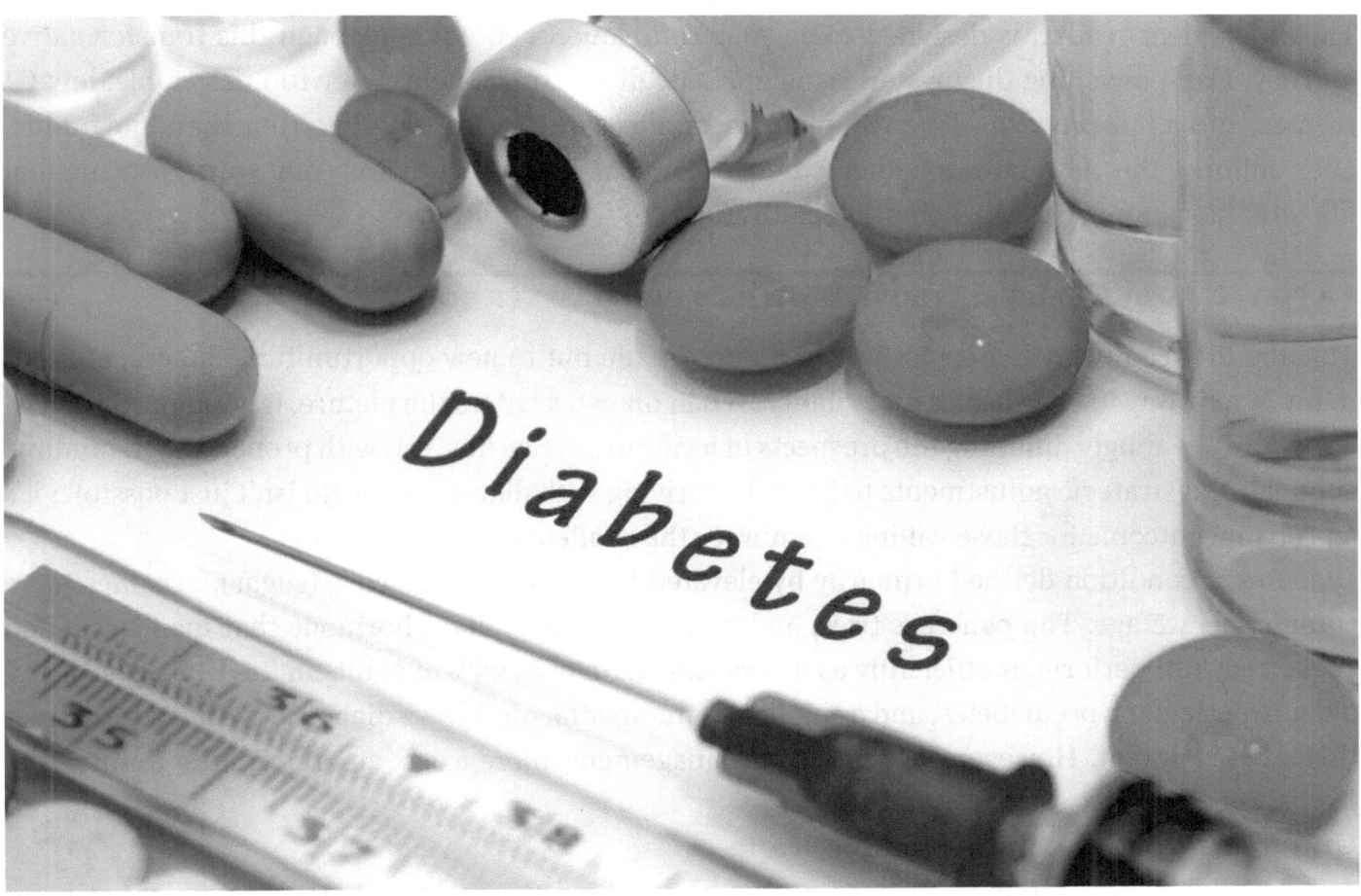

Embarking on the golden years doesn't mean dimming the vitality of life, especially for those diagnosed with diabetes after 50. It's a time marked by the richness of experience, seemingly now intertwined with a need for strict dietary vigilance. Yet, what if this period could also be an open door to revitalization and joy? Imagine mastering your health while savoring delicious meals that keep both palate and blood sugars in cheerful agreement.

Welcome to a new chapter in managing diabetes — where control aligns with culinary delight, and daily meals are crafted not just to sustain, but also to delight. The transition might seem daunting at first, akin to learning a new language at a stage when most are set in their ways. Yet, just like any profound change, it's seeded in a series of small, achievable steps.

Understanding the Low Glycemic Index (GI) approach is your first ally. This isn't merely about redefining your diet; it's about transforming it into a tool that combats the effects of diabetes while enhancing the flavors of your life. The right foods become your medications, your protectors, and your treats. They ensure the sugar level dances to a tune that promotes longevity and health.

But apart from the physical, managing diabetes is a mental and emotional marathon. It's one thing to change what's on your plate; it's another to change your mindset about food and your body. Overcoming these emotional hurdles is crucial. It fosters resilience and prepares you for this rewarding journey of self-care. It is about building a vibrant landscape from which your body and spirit can thrive, knowing well that every meal, every bite, is a step towards not just living, but thriving with diabetes.

This book, dear reader, is designed to be your companion and guide through this transformative journey. From unveiling the mysteries of a diabetic diet to introducing over 100 delectable, low-GI recipes, and a fail-proof 28-day meal plan, we aim to elevate your path to a robust and joyful life. Let's embrace this new dawn together, where each meal enriches both body and spirit, proving that life after 50 can indeed be deliciously healthy.

• A NEW CHAPTER IN LIFE: THRIVING WITH DIABETES AFTER 50

Turning fifty can open a door not just to a new decade but to new opportunities, choices, and, for many, a new way to view health and vitality. When diabetes enters the picture, it might initially cast a shadow, seemingly dimming the prospects of a vibrant, active life. Yet, with proper understanding, support, and strategic adjustments to lifestyle, thriving with diabetes post-50 isn't just possible; it's a probable outcome for those willing to embrace the challenge.

Diabetes, a condition defined primarily by elevated levels of blood glucose (sugar), becomes more common as we age. The pancreas tires, and its insulin, that valiant hormone that manages blood sugar, may not perform as efficiently as it once did. With over 33% of adults in the U.S. ages 65 and older experiencing prediabetes, and a significant number facing Type 2 diabetes, the need to address this issue is urgent. However, beyond mere management, there exists an opportunity to thrive, to transform adversity into advantage.

Understanding the Changed Landscape

At fifty and beyond, your body does not recover as swiftly, it doesn't fend off weight gain or metabolize sugar as efficiently, but it can still be molded into a haven of health with the right food and lifestyle choices. Your dietary needs shift; simplicity and moderation become paramount, and the focus on nutrient-dense, low-glycemic-index foods can turn a routine diet into a powerful delineator of health.

Embracing the Role of Diet

The role of diet becomes not just important but foundational at this stage of life with diabetes. The goal is to stabilize blood sugar levels, mitigating the daily ups and downs that can exacerbate the condition. Low-glycemic foods, which have a minimal impact on blood sugar levels, become the staples of your dietary regime. Foods like whole grains, leafy greens, most fruits, and lean proteins do not just maintain glucose levels but also satisfy nutritional needs without excessive calories.

Meeting Challenges Head-On

It's common to encounter feelings of frustration, restriction, and isolation when dietary changes become necessary. However, this new dietary journey need not be embarked upon alone. Building a supportive community, whether through in-person support groups or online forums, can greatly alleviate the mental and emotional toll of managing diabetes. Sharing experiences, recipes, and life hacks with those who understand can turn daunting roadblocks into minor hurdles.

Understanding through Education

Knowledge, especially in the form of practical, digestible information, empowers. By understanding why certain foods affect your glucose levels and how your body responds to them, you gain weapons in your arsenal against diabetes. Education on how to read and interpret nutritional labels, understanding carb counting, and realizing how different foods interact with diabetes medications are crucial skills that make the journey smoother.

Crafting a New Self-Identity

One aspect of thriving, not just surviving, with diabetes after 50 is redefining oneself in the context of this condition. You're not merely a patient; you're a fighter, a connoisseur of fine, healthy food, an explorer on a journey towards optimum health. Embrace this identity with both hands, and let it be a positive force in your life.

Real-Life Application: Success Stories

There's nothing more powerful than real-life examples to illustrate the potential for success. Consider the story of Jane, a 55-year-old former school principal. Diagnosed with Type 2 diabetes, she initially saw it as a life sentence to bland food and severe restrictions. Through nutritional education, experimenting with diverse cuisines that focus on spice rather than sugar and fat for flavor, and incorporating gentle exercise, she transformed her life. Her diabetes is not just managed; it's controlled in a way that allows her energy and vitality.

Or take Michael, a retired veteran, who turned his love for barbecue into a gourmet, diabetic-friendly art form. By tweaking traditional recipes to include sugar alternatives and more vegetables, he maintained his passion for cooking without compromising his health. His story is a testament to the fact that a diabetes diagnosis can be a gateway to innovation in the kitchen.

Concluding Thoughts

Thriving with diabetes after 50 is a confluence of diet, exercise, mental health, and community. It's about knowing your body's needs and meeting them with grace, creativity, and resilience. This isn't an end to enjoying food or fearing every meal; it's about making every dish serve your body and your taste buds equally.

Imagine carving a pathway through a dense forest. Each step, each choice makes the next one easier, eventually culminating in a trail that others can follow. That's what mastering life with diabetes after 50 entails—blazing a trail not just for yourself, but for others, proving every day that with the right attitude and tools, you can not only manage but indeed, thrive.

• UNDERSTANDING THE LOW GLYCEMIC INDEX APPROACH

Navigating the world of diets can be akin to exploring a lush, unfamiliar forest—exciting possibilities hidden amidst complexity. For those managing or newly diagnosed with diabetes after 50, the Low Glycemic Index (GI) approach may be mentioned frequently by healthcare providers. But what does it really entail, and how can it transform your perception and management of diabetes?

The Glycemic Index is essentially a ranking of carbohydrates on a scale from 0 to 100 based on how rapidly and how much they raise blood sugar levels after eating. Foods with a high GI are quickly digested and absorbed, causing a rapid rise in blood sugar levels. Conversely, low-GI foods are digested and absorbed more slowly, providing a gradual, steadier supply of energy, which can be particularly beneficial for diabetics seeking to manage their blood glucose levels more effectively.

The Science Behind Glycemic Index

At its core, the GI approach is grounded in the science of endocrinology. When you consume food, particularly carbohydrates, the body converts it to glucose, which enters the bloodstream. This rise in blood glucose triggers the pancreas to release insulin, a hormone that helps cells absorb and use glucose for energy. In individuals without diabetes, this process is smooth and regulated. However, for those with diabetes, the mechanism can be hindered, either because the pancreas does not produce enough insulin or because cells are resistant to insulin.

Therefore, understanding which foods lead to a rapid glucose increase is crucial. High-GI foods can cause blood sugar spikes, followed by rapid drops, which can lead to energy fluctuations and can be harmful over time, especially for diabetics. On the other hand, low-GI foods, which cause a slower and smaller rise in blood glucose levels, can help manage these spikes, providing more stability and less strain on the body.

Integrating Low GI Foods into Daily Life

Knowing about GI and implementing it can be like learning a new language. It begins with understanding the GI values of common foods — fruits, grains, vegetables, and sweet or starchy items. Essentially, low-GI choices include most non-starchy vegetables, most fruits, and many whole grains and legumes.

Understanding doesn't stop at knowing which foods are low in GI; it's also about how to balance foods to create a meal that overall has a lower glycemic effect. This might mean balancing a higher GI food with foods that are rich in fiber, protein, or healthy fats, as these can blunt rapid increases in blood sugar.

Lifestyle and Low GI — A Symbiotic Relationship

Adopting a low-GI diet is not just a medicinal strategy but a lifestyle change. It's about making conscious choices that align with holistic well-being. It involves not just picking the right kind of carbohydrates but also understanding portion sizes and how cooking methods can affect the GI of foods. For example, al dente pasta has a lower GI compared to softer-cooked pasta. Similarly, whole fruits have lower GI values than fruit juices.

Beyond Diabetes: The Universal Benefits of Low GI

While primarily beneficial for blood sugar management, the low-GI approach has other health benefits. These include improved cholesterol levels and heart health, better satiety, which can aid in weight management, and a reduced risk of developing type 2 diabetes for those who are currently at the prediabetes stage. Thus, adopting a low-GI diet could be seen as a preventive medicine, not just a cure.

Challenges in Transition

It's crucial to acknowledge the challenges. The adjustment period can be demanding. Old habits of meal preparation and favorite dishes might need rethinking, and the immediate gratification provided by high-GI foods can be missed initially.

Moreover, myths about the complexity or the perceived increased cost of adopting a low-GI diet often deter people. In truth, fresh produce, grains, and legumes, which are staples of low-GI diets, can be economical and accessible, and integrating them into your diet can be a creative and enjoyable culinary exploration.

Success Stories: Inspiration from Real Life

Drawing inspiration, let's look at the journeys of individuals who have embraced the low-GI approach. There's the story of Lisa, a librarian, who improved her glycemic control significantly after incorporating low-GI foods into her diet. By doing so, not only did she manage her diabetes better, she also felt more energetic and less burdened by her condition.

Then there's Roger, who after retirement, was determined not to let his diabetes manage him. By learning about and cooking low-GI meals, he not only brought his blood sugar levels under control but also rediscovered a passion for cooking. These stories underscore that managing diabetes with a low-GI diet isn't just about prevention and control; it's about transformation and joy.

Concluding Thoughts

Imagine your body as a finely tuned vehicle. The low-GI approach is about fueling it with the right kind of gasoline—not the one that burns out quickly, but the one that ensures a long, steady, and reliable ride. It's about dietary choices that don't just serve the sweet tooth but support a lifestyle where diabetes is managed effectively and healthily. This journey may require a compass to navigate initially, but once the path becomes familiar, it promises a vista of enhanced health and vitality—a true testament to living well with diabetes after 50.

• OVERCOMING THE EMOTIONAL HURDLES OF DIABETES MANAGEMENT

Navigating the emotional currents of diabetes management can be as challenging as charting a course through stormy seas. Upon diagnosis, feelings such as fear, denial, and frustration are not just common; they are natural responses to a significant life change. However, understanding and moving through these emotions with grace and resilience opens a path toward thriving with diabetes, not merely managing it.

A diagnosis of diabetes, particularly in the later stages of life, can feel like a heavy blow. It may evoke fears of dependency, changes in life's quality and length, and concern over potential complications. This emotional process mirrors grief, as it signals a loss—a loss of one's former health status and perceived freedom in life choices.

Acknowledging and Understanding Emotions

The initial step towards overcoming these emotional challenges is to acknowledge them rather than suppress them. This acknowledgment leads to better understanding and management of emotions through open conversations with family, friends, and healthcare providers. Emotional support is crucial as it provides a secure base from which individuals can tackle their diabetes management more effectively. Sharing worries and receiving reassurances can alleviate the burden and mitigate feelings of isolation or alienation.

Educating the Self and Others

Education serves as a powerful antidote to fear. Understanding diabetes and its effects bolsters confidence and reduces anxiety regarding the unknown future. This approach lights up the previously dark corners filled with 'what ifs' and replaces them with 'how tos'. However, your self-education should also extend to educating others around you. As one educates friends and family, it doesn't just adjust your own lens—it realigns your community's perceptions, fostering a supportive environment where misconceptions are replaced with empathetic understanding.

Reestablishing Control

Control over one's life can seem to slip away after a diabetes diagnosis. To reclaim it, establishing a daily routine that includes monitoring blood sugar levels, planning meals, and scheduling exercise can be empowering. Moreover, setting small, achievable goals enhances a sense of agency and accomplishment, crucial elements in combating feelings of helplessness or defeatism.

Turning Management into Empowerment

Transforming diabetes management from a chore into a personally empowering activity enhances emotional well-being. This might involve exploring and cooking new low-GI recipes or finding enjoyable physical activities that fit into your lifestyle, such as dancing, gardening, or yoga. The task becomes powerful because, through these activities, you're not solely focusing on the disease—you're enhancing your life's richness despite it.

Developing Emotional Resilience

Building resilience is key in any long-term health condition management. This involves developing a mindset that is focused on finding solutions rather than dwelling on problems. Emotional resilience can be cultivated through mindfulness practices, joining support groups, or engaging in hobbies and activities that bring joy and relaxation. Such practices help maintain a positive outlook despite the ups and downs of managing diabetes.

Facing Complications with Courage

Fear of complications can cast a long shadow over day-to-day life with diabetes. Educating oneself about the risk factors and preventive measures, and maintaining regular consultation with healthcare providers, can provide reassurance. Accept that while some factors are beyond one's control, many others can be influenced positively through active management and a healthy lifestyle.

Celebrating Small Victories

Each day brings new challenges and opportunities in the journey with diabetes. By acknowledging and celebrating each small victory—be it maintaining blood sugar levels within the target range for a week, losing a pound, or simply choosing a healthy snack over a high-sugar one—you reinforce positive behaviors and foster a sense of accomplishment.

Accepting Setbacks

Setbacks are inevitable in the management of diabetes, as in life. These moments should not be seen as failures but as learning opportunities. Analyzing what led to the setback, discussing it with a diabetes educator, and adjusting management plans are constructive ways to deal with them. This approach builds not only a robust management plan but also hardens emotional resilience against future challenges.

Renewing Purpose

Lastly, finding a purpose in life beyond diabetes management can offer profound emotional fulfillment. This might include volunteering, pursuing a new hobby, or becoming an advocate for diabetes awareness. Such engagements can provide a sense of belonging and importance, detracting from the disease's dominance in one's life.

Navigating the emotional hurdles of diabetes doesn't necessitate going it alone. Armed with understanding, supportive relationships, and strategies for adaptability, one can not only manage diabetes effectively but live a full, joyful life. Let diabetes management be a journey of continual learning and personal growth rather than a path defined by fear and restriction. The narrative of your life can still be written with hope, joy, and vibrant health as the leading themes—even with diabetes in your story.

PART I: THE ESSENTIALS OF DIABETES FOR THOSE OVER 50

CHAPTER 1. DIABETES OVERVIEW

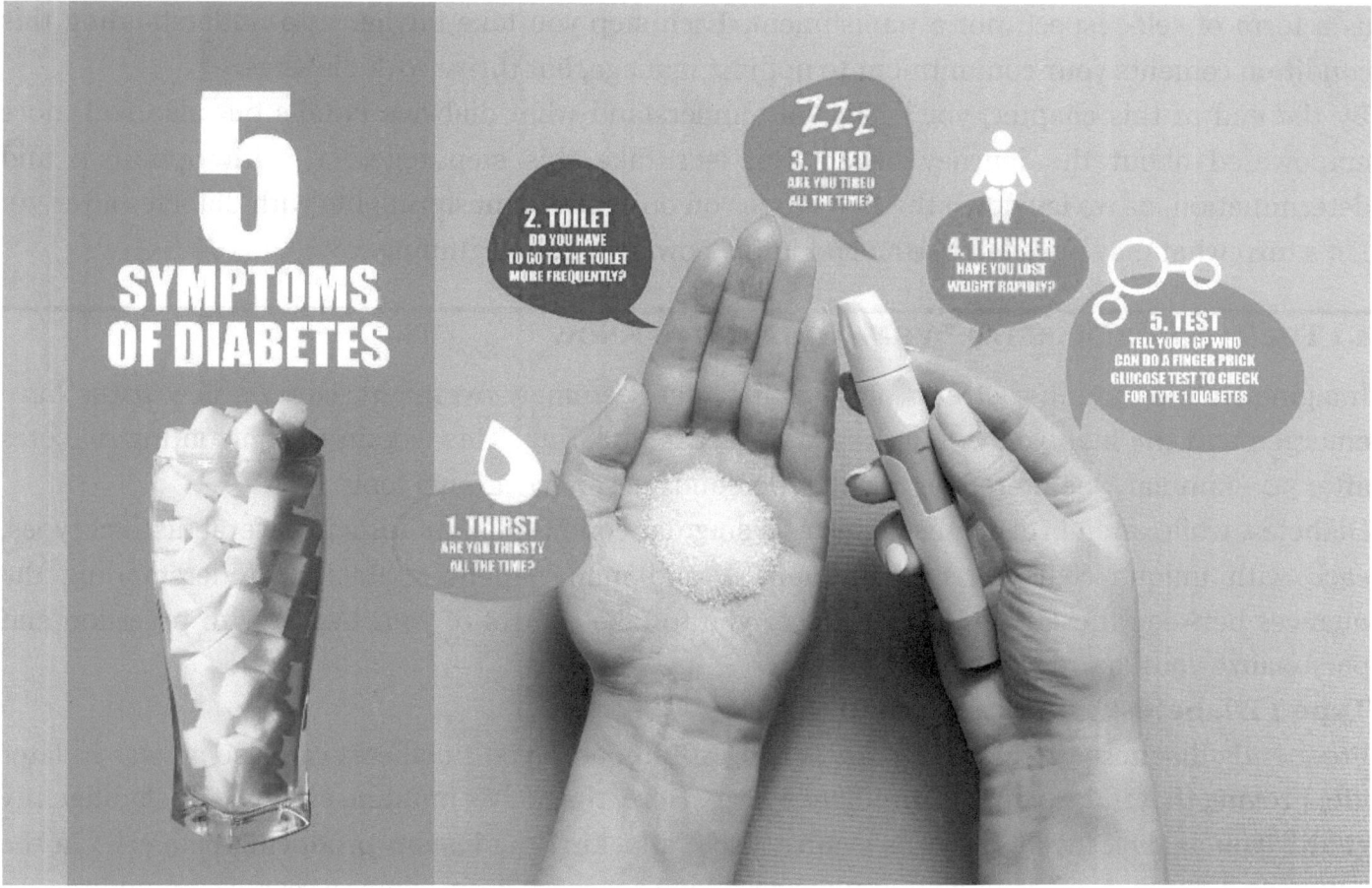

Welcome to your journey through the landscape of diabetes, particularly as you navigate the changes it brings after the age of 50. Think of this chapter as the foundation of a house we're going to build together—with each brick representing a piece of knowledge and every room a new area of understanding.

When diabetes enters our life post fifty, it often feels like a trespasser that alters the familiar landscape of our well-being. But why does it happen, and how do different types of diabetes manifest in our bodies? It might surprise you to learn that while our bodies age, our metabolic processes do too, often becoming slower and less forgiving, making us more susceptible to diabetes.

We will embark on a clear path through the types of diabetes—Type 1, Type 2, and gestational, yes, it can still be relevant at 50+! Most importantly, we'll explore how symptoms show up in subtler, sometimes misleading ways as we age. Often, a persistent thirst or a sudden change in weight might not ring alarm bells like they should. Recognizing these signs early can be the difference between a proactive or reactive approach to managing diabetes.

Moreover, knowing about diabetes is only half the battle. The other half? Understanding your body's responses. Our bodies tell stories, and symptoms are its language. By learning this language, you can become attuned to what your body needs and when it needs it.

At this stage in life, managing diabetes isn't just about adapting to dietary changes—it's about adapting to a new way of life that still promises joy and fulfillment. Think of managing your diabetes as a form of self-respect, not a punishment. Each step you take further into understanding this condition cements your commitment to not just manage, but thrive with diabetes.

By the end of this chapter, you'll not only understand what diabetes entails but also feel more empowered about the journey ahead. So, let's take this step together, with optimism and determination, as we lay down the first stones on our path to mastering life with diabetes after 50. Let's turn what may have felt like an end into a powerful new beginning.

1.1 THE TYPES OF DIABETES: WHAT YOU NEED TO KNOW

Imagine walking familiar streets only to find that seemingly overnight, curious new paths have emerged and the map you've long relied on needs updating. This is akin to confronting diabetes after 50—familiar, yet altered terrain that demands new navigational tools.

Diabetes, while often broadly discussed as a singular condition, manifests in several distinct types, each with unique characteristics, influences, and management strategies. Understanding the nuances between these types can empower you to take control of your health with precision and personalize your approach to wellness.

Type 1 Diabetes: The Unexpected Shift

Frequently diagnosed in childhood and young adulthood, Type 1 diabetes can also appear in later life, proving that it does not discriminate by age. Here, the body's immune system, which diligently guards you against invaders, turns against itself, attacking the insulin-producing beta cells in the pancreas. Insulin, the hormone that manages blood sugar levels, becomes a scarce commodity.

For those diagnosed after 50, often referred to as "LADA" (Latent Autoimmune Diabetes in Adults), the progression can be slower compared to younger Type 1 diagnoses, so the symptoms might be less obvious or mistaken for Type 2 due to age.

Type 2 Diabetes: The Gradual Onset

Type 2 diabetes constitutes the majority of diabetes cases and typically sneaks up over years. It emerges when your body starts to struggle with managing insulin efficiently—a state known as insulin resistance. Initially, your pancreas compensates by producing more insulin, but eventually, it can't keep up.

For adults over 50, the onset of Type 2 diabetes is particularly insidious because the gradual nature of its symptoms—increased thirst, frequent urination, unexplained weight changes—can be misattributed to normal aging. However, understanding these subtle hints can lead to early diagnosis and management, which is crucial in maintaining your quality of life.

Gestational Diabetes: Temporary but Telling

Primarily developing during pregnancy, gestational diabetes is a temporary condition that should be on the radar for women over 50 who are pregnant or considering pregnancy. It works similarly to Type 2, with the body failing to effectively use insulin due to the hormones produced during pregnancy. While it usually resolves after childbirth, it provides critical insights into your body's future diabetes risk.

MODY: The Genetic Undercurrent

Maturity Onset Diabetes of the Young (MODY) might sound inherently youthful, but its effects can last into later life. This less common form of diabetes is predominantly inherited and involves several gene mutations. Each type of MODY affects insulin production differently and usually doesn't involve the insulin resistance typical in Type 2 diabetes. Detection can often provide a roadmap for other family members, illuminating inherited paths that may affect them too.

Why Early Detection Matters

Identifying the type of diabetes you have is more than a medical label—it's about discovering the most effective roadmap for your health journey. Management techniques vary significantly between types. For instance, Type 1 diabetes management hinges on insulin replacement via injections or a pump, crucial for survival. In contrast, Type 2 often requires lifestyle changes, medication, and possibly insulin, depending on the disease's progression.

The Changing Needs Over Time

As we age, the management of diabetes also requires adaptation. What worked at the onset may need tweaking or complete overhauls as other elements of health evolve. Navigating diabetes after 50 means paying attention to how coexisting conditions, like hypertension or cholesterol, play into diabetes management. It's akin to conducting an orchestra where each instrument must be tuned to play harmoniously.

A Personal Experience

Think of your body as a unique ecosystem. In the same way that two seemingly similar gardens can respond differently to the same environments, so too can bodies react differently to similar treatment plans. Personalized care becomes particularly crucial as you age, ensuring that treatment recommendations accommodate your body's specific responses and needs.

Tailored Management Strategies

Diet and exercise are foundational in managing Type 2 diabetes, with a focus on controlling blood sugar levels and improving insulin sensitivity. Conversely, Type 1 diabetes requires precise monitoring of carbohydrate intake matched with insulin. MODY may require minimal intervention or a use of specific sulfonylureas depending on its subtype.

No matter the type, integrating a dietary approach that considers glycemic control is a common theme—highlighting the importance of understanding how foods affect blood sugar levels. Engaging with nutritionists who can tailor these approaches based not only on diabetes type but also on personal preferences, ensuring that your diet is not a regiment but a pleasant, sustainable aspect of life.

The Journey Ahead

Knowing your diabetes type is like having the right map for your journey. It equips you with the tools to anticipate turns and adjust your strategies accordingly. As you embrace the path of managing diabetes after 50, remember that each step you take in understanding and adapting to your diabetes type enhances your ability to navigate this condition more effectively, leading to a healthier, more vibrant life. It's a journey worth every step—for knowledge, as they say, is the most potent medicine.

1.2 HOW AGING AFFECTS DIABETES

Picture aging as a natural evolution in the narrative of life, a chapter filled with both wisdom and cautionary tales, including a deeper awareness of our health. Just as the properties of materials change with time—silver tarnishing, wood weathering—our bodies, too, undergo transformations that can affect health conditions like diabetes.

Understanding how aging impacts the development and management of diabetes is akin to adjusting our vision as our eyesight matures: essential for clarity and preventing harm. As you step into this part of life's journey, it becomes profound to engage with the ways your body now responds to this condition, significantly influenced by the aging process.

The Biological Clock and Metabolic Changes

As the years advance, the body naturally experiences a decline in metabolic rate. Metabolism, that vibrant engine processing the food into energy, begins to throttle down. This change, coupled with reduced physical activity customary in later years, contributes to decreased muscle mass and increased fat accumulation. Why does this matter for diabetes? Because muscle is more efficient at absorbing glucose than fat, a reduction in muscle mass can result in higher blood glucose levels.

Furthermore, pancreatic function, crucial in the management of insulin, also alters with age. The beta cells responsible for insulin production tend to diminish, and those remaining become less efficient in responding to blood sugar changes. Insulin resistance creeps in, silently yet impactfully, often making type 2 diabetes an uninvited guest in the lives of many aging adults.

Hormonal Adjustments

Hormones, those biochemical messengers that flick switches in nearly all body systems, also dance to a different tune as we age. For instance, amylin, a hormone that complements insulin by slowing glucose absorption and suppressing glucagon post meals, is produced less. The decrease in amylin production can exacerbate glucose control issues prevalent in elderly diabetics.

Immune System and Healing

One's immune system doesn't remain as robust as it once might have been in youth. With a reduced immune response, older adults face a higher risk of infections, which can aggravate diabetes and lead to further complications like slow healing wounds. This susceptibility makes vigilant monitoring and management of blood glucose levels even more critical.

Neurological Function and Sensory Decline

With aging, nerves might not carry messages as efficiently as before, a condition known as neuropathy, which is particularly common in people with diabetes. This condition not only causes pain and discomfort but can also result in loss of sensation, notably in extremities. Why is this significant? Because loss of sensation increases the risk of injury, which might go unnoticed and lead to complications such as ulcers or even more severe outcomes.

Furthermore, sight, crucial for managing insulin injections and monitoring glucose levels, often declines. Presbyopia, the impairment of near vision experienced by many as they age, can make reading glucose meters and insulin syringe markings challenging, increasing the risk of errors in medication.

Cognitive Aspects

Our cognitive capabilities—how we process, remember, and utilize information— can wane as we get older. For someone managing diabetes, this might manifest as forgetfulness in taking medication, missing doctor's appointments, or failing to adhere to dietary recommendations. Each of these slips, while seemingly minor, can have significant repercussions on managing diabetes effectively.

Adapting Diabetes Management to Aging

Managing diabetes in the context of aging demands an adaptive approach that accommodates these bodily changes. It may mean more frequent monitoring of blood glucose levels to counteract the increased unpredictability introduced by these aging-related changes. Dietary modifications might be necessary to adapt to altered metabolic rates and decreased energy requirements.

Moreover, education on diabetes management should be adapted to address the specific challenges aging presents. This might involve using more accessible tools for monitoring diabetes, engaging in physical activities suited to older adults that help maintain muscle mass and enhance insulin sensitivity, and adopting technologies that remind and track medication schedules.

Navigating Aging with Diabetes

Navigating the complexities of aging with diabetes is no small feat. It involves a comprehensive understanding of how aging affects bodily functions and its implications for diabetes management. It's a delicate balance, adjusting the sails as the winds of age shift and change. Armed with knowledge and the proper tools, managing diabetes in later life can become a well-charted journey rather than an uncertain voyage.

As we continue to explore diabetes management specialized for those over 50, it becomes evident that understanding these aspects of aging is not just beneficial—it's indispensable. By adjusting our approach and expectations, we can continue to live vibrant, fulfilling lives, not in spite of diabetes and aging, but in harmonious coexistence with them.

1.3 RECOGNIZING THE SYMPTOMS AND EARLY SIGNS

Embarking on a journey always requires an understanding of the signs along the road. Just as a traveler learns to read the subtle hints of a winding path or the changing weather, anyone navigating life with diabetes must become adept at recognizing its early signs and symptoms—especially as these signs often whisper quietly in the background of our busy lives.

For those over 50, diabetes can initially present as an uninvited, subtle guest, gradually making its presence known through various changes in the body. Knowing what to look for can mean catching diabetes early, greatly improving the management prospects and reducing the risk of complications.

Subtle Beginnings: Common but Overlooked Signs

One classic symptom of diabetes is an increased need to urinate. It's a direct result of the body trying to rid itself of excess glucose through urine. What makes this symptom particularly easy to dismiss in older adults is the common misconception that it's merely a factor of aging or, for men, may be chalked up to prostate problems.

Similarly, excessive thirst and increased fluid intake may seem relatively benign. Yet, when considered in relation to the other symptoms, they serve as clear indicators of the body's struggle to maintain a healthy glucose level.

Unexpected weight loss is another red flag. Despite consuming more—or at least the same amount of food—sudden weight loss might occur. This happens because diabetes prevents cells from receiving glucose, forcing the body to burn fat and muscle for energy, leading to weight loss.

The Misinterpreted Signs: Fatigue and Vision Changes

Fatigue is another symptom that those over 50 might mistakenly attribute to "just getting older" or having a busy lifestyle. However, when energy levels don't rebound with rest, it's important to consider that unmanaged diabetes may be the underlying cause.

Vision changes, too, are often misinterpreted as age-related decline. In reality, high blood sugar levels can cause fluid to be pulled from the tissues of the eyes, including the lenses, affecting the ability to focus. This can make vision temporarily blurry and should prompt consideration of blood sugar screening.

Nerve Pain and Tingling: Symptoms Not to Ignore

Diabetes can also manifest as neuropathy, wherein high sugar levels damage the nerve fibers. This condition predominantly affects the nerves in the legs and feet, leading to sensations of pain, tingling, or numbness. Often, individuals may not immediately associate these changes with diabetes, considering them instead to be symptoms of unrelated health issues like arthritis or effects of aging.

Delayed Healing: The Quiet Warning Sign

Injuries that are slow to heal, or infections that linger longer than usual, can also be potent early warnings of diabetes. High levels of glucose in the blood can eventually weaken the immune system, making it harder for the body to heal. Likewise, gum infections or other dental issues should also raise concern, as they too can be indicative of higher than normal blood sugar levels.

Recognizing Patterns: The Key to Early Identification

It's not usually one symptom alone that signals the onset of diabetes, but rather a combination or a pattern that emerges. Keeping a simple journal of health changes can help you and your healthcare provider recognize these patterns more quickly. Logging daily symptoms, diet, exercise, and even mood can reveal insights into your overall health and point to diabetes if it is indeed present.

Proactivity in Wellness: Consulting Healthcare Providers

Should these signs begin to form a pattern, the proactive step is to consult with a healthcare provider. They can perform or order tests such as the A1C test, which measures average blood glucose levels over the past three months, not just at a single moment. Such tests are invaluable in confirming whether these symptoms are indeed due to diabetes.

Lifestyle Adjustments: The First Line of Defense

Upon noticing symptoms, immediate but small lifestyle adjustments can make a significant difference. Increasing daily activity slightly, improving dietary choices, and even staying hydrated can help manage the symptoms while awaiting a definitive diagnosis. These actions are particularly important for those suspected of having prediabetes, as they can sometimes reverse the condition or prevent diabetes from developing fully.

Embracing the Significance of Early Detection

As we explore the realm of diabetes, recognizing the early signs and symptoms empowers us not only to take charge of our health but also to engage with it more deeply. Early detection is key to managing diabetes effectively and maintaining quality of life after 50. Like the wise gardener who spots the first signs of pest damage and acts swiftly to save his plants, so too must we observe and act, nurturing our health with informed, timely care.

In understanding and responding to these signs, we not only manage diabetes more effectively but embrace a proactive stance towards aging, ensuring our later years are not just about survival, but about living well.

CHAPTER 2.HEALTH IMPLICATIONS AND PREVENTION

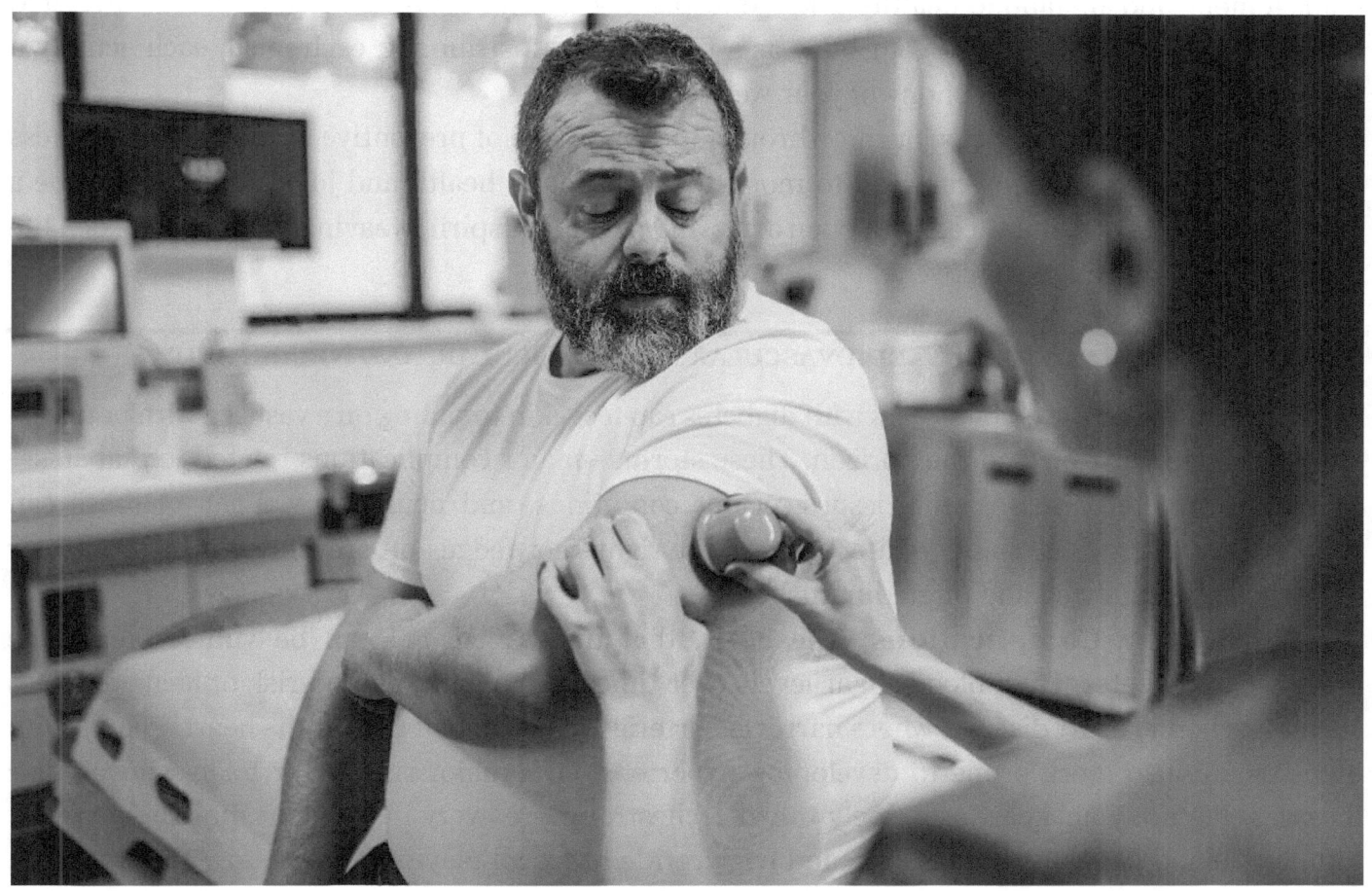

As we gracefully age beyond the 50s, our bodies narrate a complex tale of transformation, where wisdom garners more than just the silver in our hair—it touches various aspects of our health that require careful attention, particularly if living with diabetes. Embracing the wisdom of preventive care in diabetes management is akin to learning the art of balancing intricate dance steps on life's expansive stage.

Strategically navigating through the territory of health complications associated with diabetes—be it cardiovascular woes, kidney challenges, or the silent whispers of nerve damage—demands more than just a theoretical understanding. It requires a mosaic of early detection strategies, ongoing vigilance, and proactive lifestyle adjustments. Many wonder if this means a relentless pursuit of what's been lost to age. Yet, I invite you to see it as an opportunity to set a new course toward longevity and vitality.

Diabetes, while daunting, unravels a pathway that, if managed well, can transform vulnerability into strength. The longstanding belief that prevention is better than cure finds a robust echo in the corridors of aging with diabetes. Let us delve into understanding the art of recognizing signs that seek attention—a sudden blur in vision, a persistent fatigue, or perhaps, a tingling that wasn't there before. These are your body's whispers, nudging you towards early detection, which can significantly tilt the scales in your favor.

Amidst learning the ropes of managing and foreseeing symptoms, weighs the golden scale of weight management and metabolic health—a key duo playing pivotal roles in keeping diabetes-related complications at bay. Think of your body as a finely tuned instrument; each meal, each activity a note played towards the symphony of your wellbeing.

Therefore, in this chapter, let's journey through the landscape of preventive strategies and witness how small, consistent steps can lead to monumental gains in health and joy. Let health not be a pursuit but a lifestyle embraced with open arms and a resilient spirit, weaving the narrative of a life well-lived and thoroughly enjoyed.

2.1 MAJOR COMPLICATIONS: CARDIOVASCULAR, RENAL, OCULAR, AND NEUROPATHY

Navigating through the golden years with diabetes can feel akin to sailing on a vast sea with potential storms brewing just beyond the horizon. These storms—major complications related to diabetes—are cardiovascular disease, renal issues, ocular conditions, and neuropathy. Each of these can significantly affect your quality of life, but with the right knowledge and preventive measures, their impact can be managed and often diminished.

Cardiovascular Complications: The heart, that tireless engine, can be vulnerable in the presence of diabetes. High blood sugar levels over time lead to an increased risk of heart diseases such as ischemic heart disease, where narrowed arteries reduce blood flow to the heart. People with diabetes are also more prone to developing hypertension, a major risk factor for cardiovascular diseases. Picture your heart as a finely tuned orchestra where every instrument must be perfectly attuned—blood pressure, cholesterol, and triglyceride levels all playing in harmony. Disruption in this harmony leads to conditions such as atrial fibrillation, heart attacks, or strokes. The key to management lies in regular cardiovascular screening and adopting heart-healthy habits like regular physical activity, eating a balanced diet rich in fish, fruits, and vegetables, and managing stress effectively.

Renal Implications: Our kidneys, the silent sifters of our body, get no respite from their duty of filtering waste. In the presence of diabetes, these diligent workers can be overburdened, leading to diabetic nephropathy, one of the most severe complications of diabetes. Initially, there might be no symptoms as kidney damage can stealthily progress, but over time, signs such as swelling in limbs, tiredness, and altered mental alertness can signal kidney malaise. Prevention, in this case, centres around controlling blood sugar and blood pressure, regular monitoring of kidney function through tests like the ACR (albumin to creatine ratio), and potentially moderating protein intake to lessen the kidneys' workload.

Ocular Health: Imagine, if you will, the camera of your life—your eyes. Diabetes can insidiously affect these vital organs through conditions like diabetic retinopathy. The high sugar levels can cause damage to the blood vessels in the retina leading to blindness if not managed in time. Another condition, diabetic macular edema, wherein fluid accumulates in a part of the retina responsible for sharp vision, can also occur. The key to protecting your vision is regular comprehensive eye exams which can catch early changes and prevent severe visual impairment. Treatments such as laser therapy, injections, and surgery, when recommended by a specialist, can manage the progression effectively.

Neuropathy: Last but certainly not least, neuropathy or nerve damage, is a silent companion to many with diabetes. The excess sugar can injure the walls of the tiny blood vessels that nourish your nerves, especially in the legs. Symptoms can range from pain and tingling to debilitating numbness, significantly impacting the quality of life. The feet, devoid of sensation, can become prone to injury without one's immediate knowledge, leading to complications as severe as amputations. Preventive strategies involve regular foot examinations, maintaining blood sugar levels within target ranges, and wearing appropriate footwear to protect and reduce the risk of wounds.

Each of these complications carries its narratives of caution and hope. Integrating a proactive approach towards your health can make a significant difference. Regular health screenings, tailored dietary choices that respect the needs of your heart, kidneys, eyes, and nervous system, along with physical activity, can construct a formidable defense against these potential complications.

Moreover, this fight against diabetes and its associated risks isn't a solo journey. It involves collaborative care where healthcare providers, family, and community resources come together to support and empower you. It requires an understanding that, while diabetes is a part of your life's journey, it does not define it. By articulating the risks and firmly embracing preventive measures, you're not just surviving; you're thriving – turning what could be a tale of caution into one of triumph. This comprehensive strategy enhances your journey, ensuring that each step taken is robust, informed, and filled with the anticipation of a healthier future.

2.2 THE IMPORTANCE OF EARLY DETECTION AND REGULAR MONITORING

In the tapestry of managing diabetes, particularly after the age of 50, the threads of early detection and regular monitoring weave a safety net that can often mean the difference between major health upheavals and maintaining a steady course. Imagine setting off on a long voyage. Just as a seasoned captain periodically checks the integrity of his ship, reviews the weather conditions, and adjusts the sails, so too must individuals with diabetes remain vigilant in managing their condition.

Early detection in the realm of diabetes management is much like spotting a storm from afar on the horizon. It offers the crucial advantage of time and preparation. Detecting diabetes or prediabetes early can be pivotal, enabling interventions that can drastically reduce the risk of complications such as cardiovascular disease, kidney damage, and nerve problems. To understand this better, consider glucose levels as an ongoing metric that, like a thermometer, tells you the 'temperature' of your glycemic environment. Regular checks, therefore, help in maintaining the right balance, alerting you if levels begin to tip towards the extremes.

Routine monitoring includes scheduled glycemic checks, but it extends beyond this to include blood pressure measurements, cholesterol profiles, and screenings for complications. Such consistent observation is akin to the practice of tuning a musical instrument regularly to ensure it produces the right sound. For those aged 50 and above, the body's responses might not be as robust or as quick as they once were. This attenuation in physiological resilience makes regular monitoring not just good practice but an essential strategy in the proactive health maintenance toolkit.

Let's delve into what regular monitoring entails and understand its multifaceted benefits: 1. **Glycemic Control**: Regular monitoring of blood glucose levels with a glucometer provides immediate feedback on your diet, exercise, and medication's effectiveness. This real-time data allows for quick adjustments, much like a driver shifts gears instantly based on the road's incline. 2. **HbA1c Testing**: Hemoglobin A1c tests, which offer a snapshot of your average blood sugar levels over the past two to three months, should be a regular part of your health check routine. They help paint a broader picture of how well diabetes is being managed over time. 3. **Lipid Profiles**: At least once a year, it is wise to evaluate your lipid levels. This test will measure cholesterol, including LDL (bad cholesterol) and HDL (good cholesterol), and triglycerides, which are linked to the risk of cardiovascular disease. 4. **Blood Pressure**: High blood pressure, often hand-in-hand with diabetes, compounds the risk of heart disease, stroke, and kidney issues. Regular monitoring can help manage this silent threat effectively. 5. **Eye Examinations**: Comprehensive eye exams, recommended annually, can catch early signs of retinopathy, cataracts, and other ocular conditions that diabetes can exacerbate. 6. **Foot Inspections**: Daily personal checks and regular professional exams are critical as diabetes can lead to poor blood circulation and nerve damage in the feet, sometimes leading to severe infections without timely intervention.

Moreover, beyond these physical checks, regular monitoring promotes a deeper responsibility and active participation in one's health management. It fosters a habitual mindfulness about one's body and its functioning, often leading to quicker detection of irregularities and prompt medical consultation.

The psychological benefit of this regular, structured health maintenance can be substantial. It often imbues a sense of control and empowerment—key drivers in managing a chronic condition like diabetes. When people monitor regularly and see positive outcomes, it reinforces the behaviors and lifestyle changes that led to those outcomes, creating a virtuous cycle of health maintenance.

Of course, introducing such regular check-ups and tests in one's routine can initially seem daunting. Many fear that the constant reminders of their condition could add stress rather than alleviate it. Yet, with the right approach, integrating these practices can become as natural and habitual as any other daily activity, such as brushing teeth or reading the morning paper.

Thus, if there's one cornerstone habit that can amplify the effectiveness of managing diabetes after 50, it is the commitment to early detection and regular monitoring. By adopting this proactive approach, not only can the onset of diabetes-related complications be delayed, but often, their severity can be significantly reduced. The journey with diabetes is undeniably challenging, but with the compass of regular monitoring, the route becomes less perilous and a future of wellness much more attainable.

Within the constellation of factors influencing diabetes management as we age, weight management and metabolic health shine particularly brightly. It's well-documented that having a healthy weight can significantly cushion against various diseases, and for those living with diabetes after 50, it can be a profound cornerstone of daily management.

Imagine your body as a city with its own energy supply and waste management systems. When everything runs smoothly, the city thrives—buses run on time, parks stay clean, and there's less congestion. Similarly, when your weight is in a healthy range, your body manages its glucose and energy use more effectively, preventing backups and breakdowns that can escalate into major health problems.

The Symbiotic Relationship Between Weight and Diabetes

Elevated body weight, especially obesity, increases the body's resistance to insulin, demanding that the pancreas work harder to produce more insulin to lower blood sugar levels. This strain can lead to its progressive failure, exacerbating diabetes. Conversely, diabetes by itself, through its complex hormonal interactions, can make weight management more challenging. It's a cyclical relationship where managing weight can significantly alleviate the burdens of diabetes, and controlling diabetes can aid in maintaining a stable weight.

How Weight Affects Metabolic Health

Metabolic health is an umbrella term that covers various markers indicative of your overall health, including blood sugar levels, cholesterol levels, blood pressure, and waist circumference. These markers are like the vital signs of your city's health—when they're out of balance, problems loom on the horizon. For instance, excessive weight tends to skew these markers towards dangerous zones, increasing the risk not only of worsening diabetes but also of causing cardiovascular diseases, kidney problems, and more.

Strategies for Effective Weight Management

Managing weight effectively as we age requires a balanced approach that includes nutrition, physical activity, and possibly medical interventions:

1. **Nutritional Modifications**: Emphasizing a diet rich in nutrients, low in calories, and moderate in carbohydrates is crucial. Foods with a low glycemic index that do not spike blood sugar levels drastically are particularly beneficial. Fiber-rich foods, lean proteins, and healthy fats should be staples in your diet. Each meal should be a purposeful blend of these components, designed not only to satiate hunger but also to optimize your body's metabolic processes.

2. **Physical Activity**: Regular physical activity can help maintain or lose weight but is particularly effective in improving insulin sensitivity. This doesn't necessarily mean hours at the gym; even moderate, consistent activities like walking, swimming, or yoga can have significant benefits. The key is regularity and finding an activity that you enjoy, turning it from a chore into a rejuvenating part of your daily routine.

3. **Behavioral Strategies**: Sometimes, managing one's weight isn't just about knowing what to do; it's about adapting strategies to follow through consistently. Support groups, regular consultations with dietitians, and even digital tools like apps for tracking food and physical activity can play important roles in staying on course.

4. **Medical Interventions**: In some cases, medication or surgery may be recommended. These interventions are typically considered when lifestyle changes have not been sufficient, and the health risks due to excess weight are severe.

The Holistic Impact of Maintaining a Healthy Weight

Much like a well-maintained city that provides its residents with a higher quality of life, a body that is nurtured through proper weight management and metabolic control offers a robust defense against the complications of diabetes. Moreover, the psychological uplift that comes from maintaining a healthy weight and metabolism can not be overstated. It can significantly enhance quality of life, instill a sense of personal accomplishment, and equip one with the confidence to manage diabetes proactively.

Regular Monitoring: The Compass for Navigating Weight Management

Just as cities conduct regular audits and surveys to understand their functioning and prepare better for the future, regular health monitoring—in consultation with healthcare providers—can offer invaluable insights into the effectiveness of your weight management strategies. This includes regular check-ups, blood tests, and more specialized tests tailored to your personal health metrics.

In sum, as we traverse the landscape of aging, weight management and maintaining metabolic health are not just items on a checklist; they are integral to the quality of our journey. They require consistent attention, adaptability, and a proactive attitude towards one's lifestyle choices. By focusing on these areas, individuals living with diabetes can actively shape their path towards not just a longer life, but one brimming with vitality.

PART II: MASTERING YOUR DIET

CHAPTER 3. FUNDAMENTALS OF A DIABETIC DIET

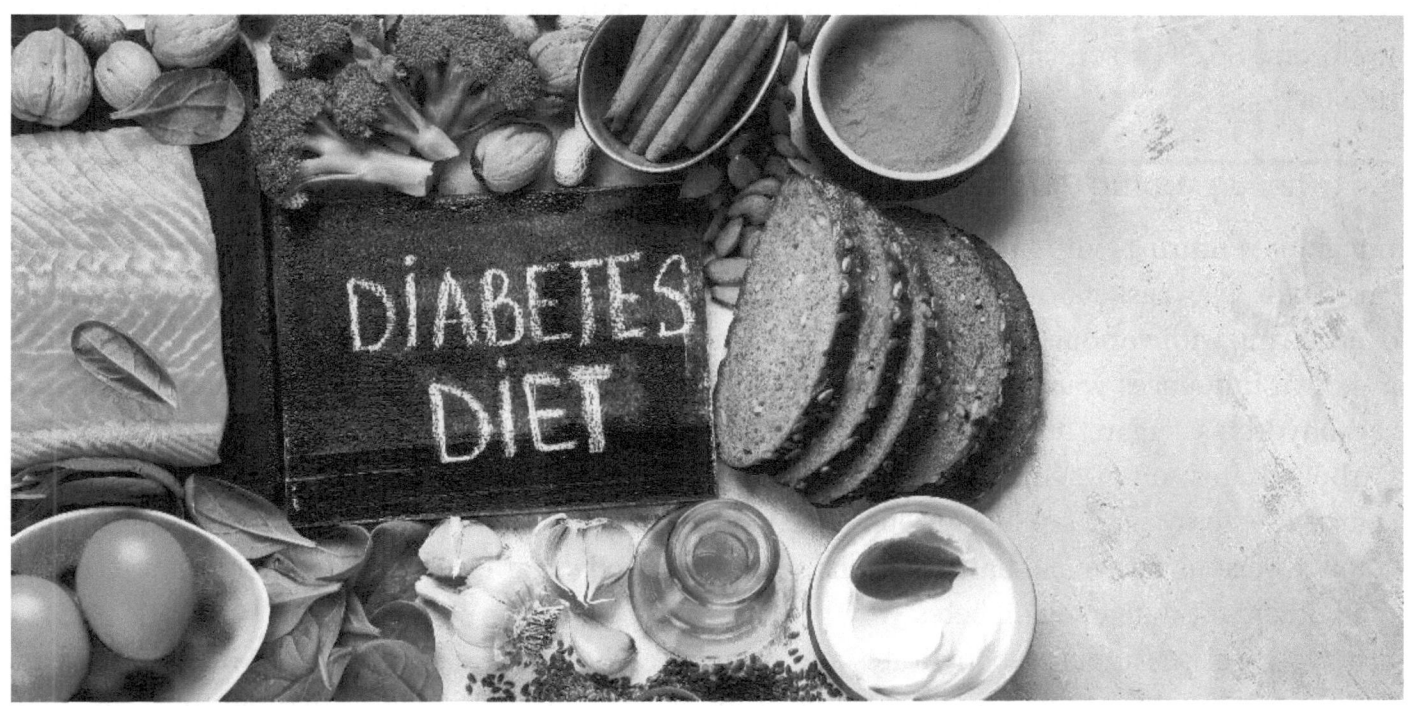

Navigating the world of food as a diabetic over fifty can sometimes feel like sailing in uncharted waters. Imagine yourself as a seasoned captain of a ship, each meal a voyage where the right supplies—an understanding of carbohydrates, proteins, and fats—are crucial not just for survival but for thriving. This chapter is your charted map to mastering your diabetic diet, a cornerstone of your health journey.

Carbohydrates have garnered quite a reputation—sometimes villainized, occasionally misunderstood. But let me assure you, it's all about types and timing. Carbs are akin to the fuel that powers your vessel; the wrong kind might steer you into turbulent waves, while the right ones keep you sailing smooth. Learning about the glycemic index will reveal how different foods affect your blood sugar, helping you choose carbs that allow you to manage your diabetes without missing out on the joys of eating.

Protein, your ship's sturdy hull, helps to stabilize blood sugar and provides essential building blocks for repair and growth. Fats, often wrongly accused rebels of the nutritional seas, are actually precious cargo. They're vital for hormone health and absorbing vitamins, yet the type of fat matters immensely. Here, we'll differentiate between those that fortify your health and those that might sabotage it.

Lastly, picturing the nutrition labels as your navigational tools is fundamental. These labels are not just small print on packaging but gateways to better understanding and choices. Deciphering them isn't just about seeing numbers and percentages—it involves understanding the impact of each component listed on your health voyage.

This chapter aims to provide you with the knowledge and confidence to make informed dietary choices that support your diabetic management. With each page, imagine us sitting together, plotting your course on a map, marking the safe harbors where you can anchor and enjoy your meals without fear or frustration. Here, we transform from mere food consumers into informed culinary explorers. So, let's set sail together, equipped and empowered, toward a horizon of health and satisfaction.

3.1 UNDERSTANDING CARBS, SUGARS, AND GLYCEMIC INDEX

Imagine venturing into a grand market where the aisles are lined with myriad forms of carbohydrates: baskets of colorful fruits, shelves brimming with all manners of bread, and bins overflowing with various grains and legumes. Each of these foods carries its own story, particularly in how it influences your blood sugar levels. To navigate this expanse wisely, an understanding of carbohydrates, sugars, and the glycemic index is indispensable.

Carbohydrates, often simply called carbs, are one of the primary macronutrients and the main source of energy in many diets around the world. However, not all carbs are created equal. They come in various forms and have different effects on blood sugar levels, making some choices better than others for managing diabetes.

Firstly, there are simple carbohydrates and complex carbohydrates. Simple carbs, including sugars like glucose, fructose, and sucrose, are quickly absorbed by the body, leading to rapid spikes in blood sugar. These are the sugars you find abundantly in sodas, desserts, and processed snacks—the kind of fleeting visitors in your bloodstream that cause chaos only to leave you tired and hungry. On the other hand, complex carbohydrates, such as those found in whole grains, legumes, and vegetables, are composed of long chains of sugar molecules that are slowly broken down and absorbed, providing a steadier source of energy.

Now, let's delve deeper into sugars. Sugars are ubiquitous in both naturally occurring and added forms. While fruits do contain sugar, they also offer fiber, vitamins, and minerals, making their overall impact on blood sugar more balanced. Contrast this with added sugars found in many processed foods; devoid of nutrients, they contribute to rapid glucose spikes and are, thus, a less favorable choice for blood sugar management.

This brings us to an invaluable tool for understanding our carbohydrate choices: the glycemic index (GI). The GI measures how much a specific food increases blood sugar levels compared to pure glucose, which has a GI of 100. Foods are ranked on a scale of 0 to 100, with higher values indicating a greater impact on blood sugar. For instance, a ripe banana might have a GI of around 62, whereas barley could be as low as 25. This system helps in visualizing the effect different foods can have and supports better decision-making when planning meals.

Managing diabetes is akin to being a master painter; just as an artist uses a palette to blend colors, you use the glycemic index to blend foods. Pairing a high GI food with foods lower on the index can balance the overall glycemic load of a meal. Think of a meal where a small portion of mashed potatoes, a high GI food, is balanced with leafy greens and lean protein. This combination can help mitigate rapid blood sugar increases while providing nutritional balance.

Understanding the nuances of the glycemic index also underpins the concept of glycemic load (GL). While the GI offers a measure of quality, GL quantifies quantity. It considers the GI of a food in addition to the amount of carbohydrate it contains in a typical serving, giving a fuller picture of how this food might affect blood sugar levels when actually eaten. For example, watermelon has a high GI but a low GL because the actual amount of carbohydrates in a normal serving is quite low.

Why does this matter? Because real-life eating patterns are more complex than isolated food choices. Integrating the concepts of GI and GL empowers you to craft meals that not only delight your palate but also harmonize with your body's needs, promoting an even energy flow.

Thus, embarking on a diet cognizant of the GI and GL requires not just knowledge, but also strategy. It's about more than avoiding sugar; it's about creating a mosaic of meals where each piece supports balanced blood sugar levels. Transitioning to this approach may seem daunting at first glance, but it becomes more intuitive over time. It's about making small adjustments that collectively transform how you eat.

By now, you might be wondering how all this information translates into daily decision-making. Here's the essence: opt for whole, unprocessed foods when possible; integrate plenty of fiber through vegetables, fruits, and whole grains; moderate your intake of high GI foods by pairing them with lower GI alternatives; and, above all, monitor how different foods affect your own blood sugar by using a glucose meter. After all, each person's response can vary, making personalized insights invaluable.

As we journey through the realms of carbohydrates and sugars, equipped with the compass of the glycemic index, the landscape of food becomes not just manageable but a space of empowerment. With this knowledge, you can choose foods that sustain energy levels, manage blood sugar, and support overall health, transforming the daily act of eating from a challenge into an art form that enhances your life and well-being.

3.2 THE ROLE OF PROTEIN AND HEALTHY FATS

In the tapestry of a well-rounded diabetic diet, protein and healthy fats are the threads that provide strength and texture, playing pivotal roles that extend far beyond simply satisfying hunger. Understanding the significance of these macronutrients can transform your approach to daily eating, helping you manage your diabetes with greater ease and assurance.

Proteins are like the building blocks of life, integral in forming everything from enzymes and hormones to muscles and skin. For those managing diabetes, protein's primary boon is its minimal impact on blood glucose levels. Unlike carbohydrates, proteins do not cause sudden spikes in blood sugar, thus providing a stable energy source.

The power of protein in a diabetic diet also lies in its ability to satiate hunger effectively. Consuming protein-rich foods can lead to a feeling of fullness that lasts longer than one experiences from fats or carbohydrates. This can help control overall calorie intake, which is crucial for weight management — a key factor in managing Type 2 diabetes.

However, the source of protein is just as important as the quantity. Lean meats such as chicken, turkey, and fish are excellent sources, delivering high-quality protein without the excess fats that accompany some cuts of red meats. Plant-based proteins—like lentils, beans, and quinoa—not only offer protein but also bring fiber and other nutrients to the table without the cholesterol and saturated fats found in animal proteins. This makes them a wholesome choice for anyone, especially those over 50 looking to manage heart health along with diabetes.

On the other hand, healthy fats play an equally crucial role. Gone are the days when all fats were vilified. Today, we understand that certain fats are not only permissible but essential for good health. These fats, particularly unsaturated fats, support numerous bodily functions, including the absorption of vitamins and the regulation of hormones.

Monounsaturated and polyunsaturated fats, found in olive oil, nuts, seeds, and fish, can improve blood cholesterol levels, thereby decreasing the risk of heart disease. Omega-3 fatty acids, a type of polyunsaturated fat found abundantly in fish like salmon and trout, are especially beneficial for cardiovascular health, which is often a concern for those with diabetes.

Including healthy fats in your diet can also moderate blood sugar spikes. By slowing the absorption process of carbohydrates, fats help in maintaining steadier glucose levels, providing more consistent energy throughout the day.

However, it's crucial to distinguish these beneficial fats from saturated fats and trans fats — often found in processed foods, these fats can exacerbate heart risks and other health issues. Therefore, the integration of healthy fats into the diet must be balanced with mindful avoidance of harmful fats to not counteract their health benefits.

Yet, integrating protein and healthy fats into your diet should be more about adding diversity and enjoyment than about strict restrictions. Think about marinating a piece of fish in herbs and olive oil or tossing a salad with avocado and walnuts. These are not just dietary recommendations but are invitations to explore new textures and flavors, making meals not only nutritious but also delightful.

It's also worth recognizing the synergy between protein, fats, and carbohydrates. A meal that includes all three macronutrients can help stabilize blood sugar levels better than a meal skewed heavily towards any single macronutrient. For instance, a balanced breakfast might feature a spinach and feta omelet with a side of whole-grain toast, combining protein, healthy fats, and complex carbohydrates.

Moreover, it's important for those living with diabetes and especially for those aged over fifty, to consult healthcare providers to tailor their protein and fat intake to their specific health needs. Factors such as kidney function might necessitate adjustments in protein consumption, just as cardiac concerns might influence the types of fats one should prioritize.

Addressing diabetes after 50 doesn't just involve understanding what you eat; it revolves around adopting a holistic perspective that respects how various nutrients interact within your body. It's about crafting a dietary pattern that not only keeps blood sugar levels in check but also supports overall vitality and well-being.

Thus, in the journey of managing diabetes, envision protein as your steady companion, offering lasting energy without the glycemic impact, and healthy fats as the guardians of your cellular health and satiety. Embracing these macronutrients within the thoughtful framework of a balanced diet can make the path toward health not just successful, but also enjoyable and deeply satisfying.

3.3 HOW TO READ AND INTERPRET FOOD LABELS

Entering a grocery store is akin to setting out on a treasure hunt. Every aisle and shelf holds potential gems that can enhance your diabetic diet. However, hidden among these treasures are pitfalls—foods that may seem benign but could disrupt your blood sugar management. This is where the art of reading food labels becomes crucial, transforming you from a casual shopper into an informed consumer, adept at navigating the nutritional nuances each product offers.

Food labels, however abstract they might appear initially, are essentially a dialogue between you and the manufacturer. They provide insights into what's inside the package so you can make choices aligned with your health goals. This narrative journey isn't just about avoiding what's bad, but actively seeking what's beneficial. Here is how you can become fluent in the language of food labels.

Start with the Serving Size: Every nutritional fact is related to a specific serving size. This figure forms the foundation of your interpretation. It can be tempting to overlook this detail but remember, if the serving size is one cup and you consume two, you're doubling not just your portions but also your intake of sugars, fats, and calories. Being aware of the serving size helps maintain portions that align with your dietary needs.

Understand Calories: Calories measure how much energy you get from a serving of the food. While managing diabetes, it's not just about counting calories but understanding the source of these calories—whether they come from carbohydrates, fats, or proteins—and how they fit into your overall dietary plan.

Carbs, and More Importantly, Types of Carbs: Total carbohydrates on labels include starches, fibers, and sugars. For a diabetic diet, observing the amount of fiber and sugars is vital because they impact blood sugar differently. High-fiber foods are beneficial as they help slow down glucose absorption and maintain blood sugar levels. Sugars, on the other hand, require more scrutiny. Look beyond the total sugars; check ingredients for added sugars which can spike blood sugar levels unnecessary.

Spot the Sugars: Added sugars can appear under many names – sucrose, glucose, high fructose corn syrup, and more. They can sneak into foods where you least expect them, like salad dressings or bread. Learning these terms helps in identifying products that are healthier for your blood sugar control.

Protein - Your Ally in Balance: Protein content is also listed on food labels and is essential for building and repairing tissues and playing a part in blood sugar stabilization. Diets balanced with healthy proteins can mitigate the quick absorption of sugars, aiding in overall glucose stability.

Fats - Choose Wisely: Not all fats are created equal. Labels break them down into saturated, unsaturated, and trans fats. For a heart-healthy diabetic diet, focus on foods low in saturated fats and trans fats. These fats are linked to heart disease and should be minimized. Instead, seek out products with healthier fats like mono and polyunsaturated fats, which support your heart health.

Sodium - A Sneaky Element: Sodium doesn't affect blood sugar directly but is crucial for overall health, particularly in blood pressure management. Many processed foods are high in sodium, which can lead to hypertension, a common companion to diabetes. Monitoring sodium intake is a preventative measure against cardiovascular complications.

Ingredients List - The Revealer: The list of ingredients often tells more about a product than the rest of the label. Ingredients are listed by quantity, from highest to lowest. This list can reveal added sugars, unnecessary fillers, and artificial additives that might best be avoided. It's a tool for detecting how processed a food is - the shorter the list, generally, the better.

Check for Dietary Fiber: Foods high in dietary fiber can have a significant role in a diabetic diet. High-fiber foods can help control blood sugar levels, aid digestion, and keep you feeling fuller longer, which helps in weight management. Check labels for high fiber content, particularly in cereals, bread, and pasta.

Label reading, while technical, is also a narrative about what's entering your body. Think of it as a map that guides you through the dietary choices that shape your diabetes management. It might look daunting at first glance, but with practice, label reading becomes second nature—a powerful tool in your toolkit for maintaining not just healthy glucose levels but overall vitality.

Navigating food labels effectively demands a shift from passive consumption to engaged, informed decision-making. Each label read, each ingredient list scrutinized, adds to your growing expertise in managing your diet, transforming grocery shopping from a routine chore into an empowered act of self-care. Remember, knowledge here is more than power; it is prevention, management, and above all, a pathway to better health.

CHAPTER 4. CHOOSING THE RIGHT FOODS

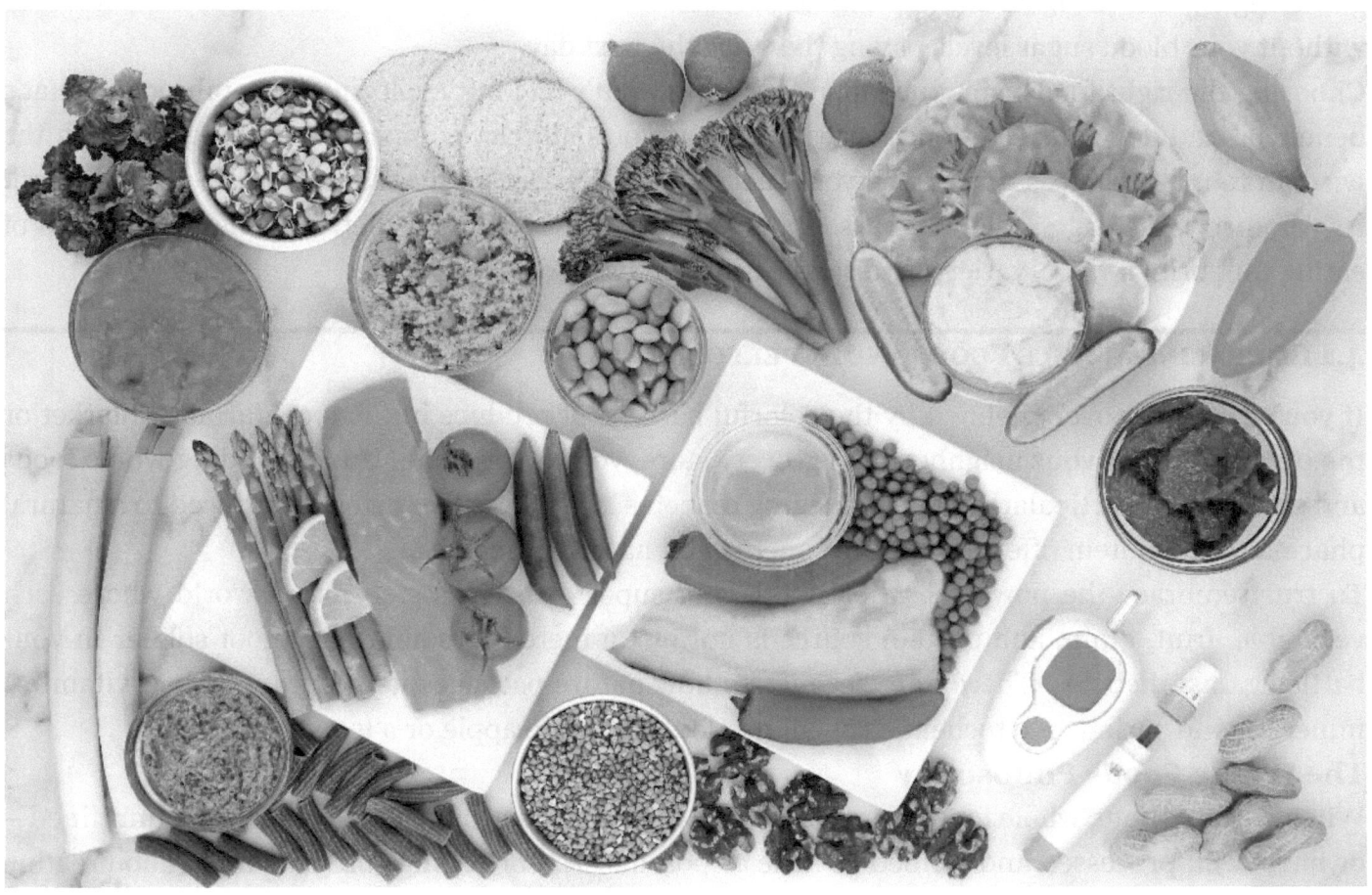

Imagine walking into your favorite grocery store, armed not just with a shopping list but with a newfound foresight—envisioning foods that heal, protect, and nourish your aging body while keeping your blood sugar levels perfectly balanced. Mastering the art of choosing the right foods is akin to learning a new language in your pursuit of a healthy lifestyle, particularly with diabetes on board as you stride past 50. It's both an art and a science, intertwining knowledge with personal experience to create a joyful, wholesome eating experience.

In this essential chapter of our journey together, we will transcend the typical drill of "dos and don'ts" and dwell on a richer understanding of food choices that cater not just to your medical needs but to your palate's pleasures as well. Each food item you choose carries a powerful potential, contributing to your overall metabolic health or detracting from it. It's crucial, therefore, to make enlightened choices.

We will start by exploring whole foods and superfoods—yes, the champions of a diabetic-friendly pantry. These are your trusty allies in stabilizing blood sugar and fending off the hungry calls of snacking on less wholesome options. But what about sweet cravings, you ask? We'll delve into that, comparing the pros and cons of natural versus artificial sweeteners and how to reconcile your sweet tooth with your health goals.

And then there's the social aspect of eating—beverages and alcohols are often at the center of gatherings. We'll navigate together through choices that allow you to toast on special occasions without your blood sugar levels paying the price the next day.

Choosing the right foods isn't only about avoiding what's bad but exploring and embracing what's beneficial and delicious. This chapter will serve as your culinary compass, equipping you with the wisdom to make choices that enrich your diet in ways that are both satisfying and health-forward. As you turn these pages, picture yourself mastering not just a diabetic diet, but a new dimension of eating that brings vigor, variety, and satisfaction into your day-to-day life.

4.1 EMBRACING WHOLE FOODS AND SUPERFOODS

If you've ever felt overwhelmed by the colorful barrage of produce in the local farmers' market or the organic aisle of your neighborhood grocery store, you're not alone. Understanding whole foods and superfoods, particularly when managing diabetes after 50, is like being introduced to a natural pharmacy—each item offering specific benefits and natural remedies.

To truly embrace the power of whole foods and superfoods, let's step into a world where each vegetable, fruit, grain, and protein source is not just a mere ingredient but a foot soldier in your battle against diabetes. There's an elegance to how nature packages its solutions—fiber, vitamins, minerals, and various phytochemicals—all nestled in a single apple or a leaf of kale.

The Whole Foods Philosophy

When we talk about 'whole foods', we're referring to foods that remain unprocessed and unrefined—or have been processed and refined as little as possible—before being consumed. It's about eating an apple instead of drinking apple juice or choosing whole grains instead of refined grains. These foods are foundational in a diabetic diet because they digest more slowly, causing a lower and slower rise in blood glucose.

Whole foods also richly supply our bodies with solvable and insoluble fibers. Solvable fibers help control blood glucose levels and lower blood cholesterol—a concern particularly pertinent as we age. Insoluble fibers, on the other hand, help food move through your digestive system, reducing the risk of constipation and improving intestinal health.

Superfoods: What's in a Name?

The term 'superfood' might sound like modern marketing jargon, but it's simply a way to describe foods exceptionally dense in nutrients—essential vitamins, minerals, antioxidants, and more—that can significantly impact your health. These are the foods that can aid weight management, reduce inflammation, and help control blood sugar levels, all crucial aspects when managing diabetes.

Let's consider, for instance, the humble blueberry. Rich in antioxidants and Phyto flavonoids, these berries are also high in potassium and vitamin C. Not only can they lower your risk of heart disease and cancer, but they have anti-inflammatory properties, which is vital in controlling chronic conditions such as diabetes.

Integrating Whole Foods and Superfoods into Your Diet

To start integrating more whole foods and superfoods into your diet, envision your plate as a canvas, half of which you'll paint with fruits and vegetables. A quarter should be whole grains—such as quinoa, brown rice, or whole grain pasta—while the final quarter is for lean protein sources, whether animal or plant-based.

Fruits and Vegetables

For fruits, focus on low glycemic index choices like cherries, grapefruits, pears—which have the double advantage of controlling your blood sugar and providing essential nutrients. Vegetables, especially non-starchy types like spinach, kale, and bell peppers, are not just low in carbohydrates but high in fiber and packed with nutrition.

Grains

In grains, shift from refined products like white bread to the nutrient-dense realms of barley, whole wheat, and rolled oats. These whole grains help in maintaining consistent blood sugar levels and contribute to your feeling of fullness during meals.

Protein

On the protein quarter of your plate, salmon—an undeniable superfood—brings omega-3 fatty acids to your table, essential for cardiovascular health, an important consideration given diabetes' impact on heart disease risk.

The Art of Substitution

One of the simplest strategies in your transition to a whole foods and superfoods diet is the art of substitution. Start with replacing one meal's refined components with whole food options. If morning finds you with a bowl of refined cereal, switch it out for oatmeal topped with a fresh blueberry compote.

Local and Seasonal: A Better Approach to Superfoods

Where possible, choose local and seasonal produce. These options are often fresher and more nutrient-dense as they are sold shortly after harvest. They are also a great way to support local farmers and reduce environmental impact, ensuring that healthy eating and environmental consciousness go hand in hand.

The Cautionary Tale of Superfoods

While superfoods are powerful allies, moderation remains key. Over-relying on them can lead to an unbalanced diet, missing out on other crucial nutrients. Diversity in your diet is just as important as the inclusion of nutrient-rich superfoods. Think of it as conducting an orchestra—while the superfoods may be the leading violin, other foods contribute equally to the symphony.

In conclusion, embracing whole foods and superfoods isn't just a dietary choice but a lifestyle decision that influences not only your physical health but also your environmental footprint. As you age, these food choices offer a pathway not just towards managing diabetes but towards a revitalized life where food is both medicine and joy. As we transition through life's later chapters, let these foods be your natural, healthful companions on a journey towards wellness and vitality.

Navigating the world of sweeteners can feel like deciphering a complex map with many routes, each claiming to be the best way to reach your destination of healthy living, especially when managing diabetes. When sugar is on the blacklist, what alternatives do we have for that sweet taste we often crave? Natural alternatives and artificial options abound, each with its pros and cons, each serving different needs and preferences. Understanding these can help blend sweetness into your life without the bitter side effects on your blood glucose levels.

The Sweet Deception - A Primer on Sugar

Firstly, it's essential to understand our main adversary in the context of diabetes - sugar. Sugar is a carbohydrate that the body converts into glucose, which raises blood sugar levels. It's not just about the white granulated sugar you might sprinkle over cereal or stir into coffee; it's also about hidden sugars in processed foods, fruit juices, and even so-called 'healthy' snacks.

Art of Substitution - Natural Sweeteners

There's a charm in using natural alternatives. They come from natural sources and undergo less processing. They often retain nutrients found in those natural sources, making them a potentially healthier choice.

Honey and Maple Syrup: Both are popular natural sweeteners but come with higher calorie counts and should be used sparingly. However, they offer antioxidants and nutrients absent in refined sugar. The key lies in their minimal use, where even a small amount can provide a significant sweetness due to their rich flavors.

Stevia: A sweetener derived from the leaves of the Stevia rebaudiana plant, stevia is many times sweeter than sugar yet has negligible effects on blood glucose levels, making it a favorite amongst those managing diabetes. It's important, however, to choose versions that are pure and not mixed with other high glycemic fillers.

Monk Fruit Sweetener: Derived from the monk fruit, a native fruit of Southeast Asia, this sweetener is another excellent natural alternative. It neither raises blood sugar nor calorie levels but shares a common downside with stevia - its aftertaste, which some might find unpleasant.

Synthetic Saviors - Artificial Sweeteners

On the other side of our map, we find artificial sweeteners, synthesized compounds designed to sweeten with fewer calories and less impact on blood sugar levels than regular sugar.

Aspartame: Commonly found in diet sodas and reduced-calorie foods. It's suitable for reducing sugar content but should be avoided by those with phenylketonuria, a rare genetic disorder, as it contains phenylalanine.

Sucralose: Known widely by its brand name, Splenda, sucralose is made from sugar but is many times sweeter and has little to no effect on blood glucose levels. It's versatile in that it can be used both in cooking and baking.

Saccharin: One of the oldest artificial sweeteners, found in products like Sweet'N Low, saccharin can be useful for diabetes management but may leave a metallic aftertaste.

Balancing Act - Combining Sweeteners

Sometimes, the key to using sweeteners effectively lies in the combination—mixing natural and artificial sweeteners to reduce the amount of each and ideally balance taste with health benefits. For instance, pairing a small amount of honey with stevia can help mitigate stevia's aftertaste while enjoying honey's flavor and minimizing its impact on blood sugar.

Impact Beyond Taste - Glycemic Response and Health

While exploring sweeteners, it's crucial not to focus solely on taste but also on the body's glycemic response. The ideal choice for managing diabetes would be sweeteners that provide the sweetness needed without causing a spike in blood glucose levels. Both the quantity and type of sweetener are vital factors in this delicate balance.

Sweeteners in Everyday Life - Practical Uses

Implementing these sweeteners into your diet isn't just about swapping sugar in your morning coffee. Consider their uses across your cooking and baking endeavors. For example, using apple sauce or mashed bananas can add natural sweetness to baked goods while providing extra nutrients and fiber.

Cautionary Notes - Potential Downsides

Despite the benefits, it's important to use sweeteners—natural or artificial—with caution. Over-reliance on sweet-tasting food, even if low in calories or carbohydrates, can maintain a craving for sugary foods, making dietary management more challenging. Additionally, some artificial sweeteners could potentially have laxative effects or cause allergic reactions in susceptible individuals.

In conclusion, understanding the nuances of sweeteners—both natural and artificial—offers a powerful toolkit for managing diabetes effectively. Being informed and mindful about each option helps maintain a healthy dietary balance, allowing the sweetness of life to flourish without compromising blood sugar management. Navigating this landscape is an ongoing journey of taste and health, one where moderation and informed choices lead the way.

4.3 ALCOHOL, BEVERAGES, AND THEIR IMPACT ON BLOOD SUGAR

Navigating the world of beverages as an individual over 50 with diabetes entails more than just choosing between diet soda and regular, or red wine and white. It requires a nuanced understanding of how different beverages can affect blood sugar levels, overall hydration, and wellness. Here, we take an insightful stroll through the effects of various drinks on our bodies, and how best to enjoy them without derailing our diabetic management plans.

Drinking—whether it's a sip of water, a gulp of beer, or a cocktail at happy hour—forms part of our everyday rituals. Each choice carries implications for blood sugar management and overall health that cannot be ignored, especially in the later stages of life when the body's response to sugar and alcohol changes.

The Case of Alcohol: Risks and Moderation

Alcohol's impact on blood sugar is paradoxically dual. While moderate alcohol consumption can cause blood sugar to rise, excessive alcohol can conversely lead to dangerously low blood sugar levels, especially if consumed on an empty stomach or when insulin or insulin promoter drugs are in play. This is due to alcohol's ability to inhibit the liver's ability to produce glucose.

Consider a common scenario: a gathering where wine flows freely. While it might seem harmless to partake in a couple of glasses, it's vital to understand that even red wine, often lauded for its health benefits due to its antioxidant properties, contains sugars that can affect your glucose control. Moderation is crucial, and so is knowledge—dry wines typically have fewer sugars than their sweeter counterparts.

The World of Coffee and Tea: Benefits with Boundaries

Coffee and tea, the stalwarts of morning rituals, also have a role to play in blood sugar management. While straight black coffee or herbal teas can potentially have minimal impact on blood sugar levels, the devil lurks in the details—or rather, in the add-ons. Sugars, creamers, and flavored syrups can quickly escalate a zero-calorie cup to a sugary concoction that spikes blood sugar levels.

Interestingly, studies have suggested that ingredients in coffee and some types of tea might actually help improve insulin sensitivity and reduce inflammation. The key, however, lies in consumption with minimal additives. Embracing these beverages in their simplest forms can be an enjoyable way to maintain hydration without risking sugar spikes.

Soft Drinks, Diet Sodas, and Artificial Sweeteners

The allure of soft drinks—with their fizz and tang—can be hard to resist. Yet, for an individual managing diabetes, regular soft drinks, laden with high amounts of fast-digesting sugars, pose a significant threat to effective glucose control. Here enters diet soda, a popular alternative touted to offer all the soda joy without the sugar rush. But caution is advised. Diet sodas often contain artificial sweeteners which can still trigger insulin, despite them not raising blood sugar in the traditional sense. Furthermore, some studies suggest potential links between frequent consumption of artificially sweetened beverages and an increased risk of metabolic syndrome and type 2 diabetes.

Fruit Juices: Natural but Not Harmless

The natural aura that surrounds fruit juice can often be misleading. Yes, these juices come from fruit, but in the juicing process, fiber is lost, and sugars become concentrated, which can lead to significant blood sugar spikes when consumed. Like with wine, moderation and portion control are key. Opting for whole fruit instead of juice offers the natural fiber of the fruit, which aids in slowing down the absorption of sugar, thus maintaining more stable blood sugar levels.

Water: The Underrated Hero

In the conversation about beverages, it's easy to overlook the simplest yet most beneficial drink—water. Water is essential for overall health and plays a critical role in helping manage blood sugar levels. It aids in diluting the blood, which can help manage high blood sugar levels. Staying well-hydrated is paramount, especially in the management of diabetes, where dehydration can be a common side effect due to elevated blood sugar levels leading to frequent urination.

Herbal Choices: A Soothing Alternative

Incorporating herbal drinks like chamomile, peppermint, or ginger tea can be a soothing, flavorful way to maintain hydration without impacting blood sugar levels. These beverages can offer calming benefits, aid digestion, and provide a comforting ritual that doesn't compromise diabetic health goals.

Concluding Sips

Understanding and managing the impact of various beverages on blood sugar levels requires a responsive and informed approach. Each drink consumed should be considered in the broader context of daily fluid and nutritional intake. Integrate beverages into your diet that complement and support your health needs rather than conflict with them.

In managing diabetes, especially after 50, the focus should always lean towards maintaining a balanced and mindful approach to eating and drinking. This ensures that life's pleasures, like a good drink, remain a part of your lifestyle without detrimental effects on your health.

CHAPTER 5. CREATING A BALANCED MEAL PLAN

Navigating your dietary needs after 50, especially with diabetes, can sometimes feel like trying to solve a complex puzzle with pieces that don't quite seem to fit. That's where the magic of crafting a balanced meal plan comes into play—an art form I'm excited to guide you through. Imagine walking into your kitchen, each shelf and drawer strategically stocked, with ingredients that promise not only nourishment but pleasure. It's entirely possible, and I'll show you how to turn this dream into your daily reality.

First, let's debunk a myth: a diabetes-friendly diet isn't about restrictions; it's about balance and making informed choices. A well-structured meal plan is not your dietary gatekeeper but your passport to a world of flavors. This chapter is dedicated to teaching you to measure the perfect portions, mix the right ingredients, and manage your meals over the course of a typical day—all while keeping those blood sugar levels in check.

Envision your meal plan as a finely-tuned orchestra where each food group plays a crucial role, yet none overpower another. Carbohydrates, proteins, and fats will harmonize to create symphonies of flavors that are as satisfying as they are healthy. And yes, the concern about bland diabetic recipes? I assure you, it's a thing of the past with the recipes and insights we'll explore here.

I will walk you through constructing a 28-day meal plan that isn't just practical but also customizable to fit into various lifestyles and preferences. Whether you're a social butterfly, hosting family gatherings, or prefer a quiet meal at home, your meal plan can be tailored to encompass all these scenarios. Imagine never again being at a loss at what to cook, eat, or serve!

Forging ahead with our culinary journey, I will guide your step by one flavorful step, ensuring every meal enriches both your body and spirit. We're not just managing diabetes; we're embracing a lifestyle that accommodates festive dinners, casual brunches, and everything in between with gusto and confidence. So, grab your apron, and let's begin this delicious, healthful adventure together.

5.1 PORTION CONTROL AND SERVING SIZES

As the gentle art of cooking permeates our daily routines, one often overlooked yet critical aspect is the mastery of portion control and understanding serving sizes. Think of it as the bridge that connects the nutritional content of food to your individual health needs, especially pivotal when managing diabetes after 50. This balance is not merely about measuring or weighing food but is rooted deeply in a philosophy that harmonizes health with pleasure without succumbing to deprivation. It's about eating right, not less, and ensuring what lands on your plate promotes your well-being.

The Art of Portion Control

The journey into mastering portion control begins with visualizing what a balanced plate looks like. Imagine your favorite painting. What makes it a masterpiece? Is it not the balance of colors, the proportion of elements, each contributing uniquely to a harmonious outcome? In much the same way, your meal plate is your canvas, and your food choices the colors with which you paint. To start, visualize your plate divided into sections: half of it filled with a riot of colorful vegetables, a quarter with lean protein, and the remaining quarter with whole grains or starchy vegetables. This visual guide helps create meals that are satisfying yet balanced in nutrients that keep your blood sugar levels steady.

Adjusting portions can feel daunting at first glance. The fear of ending up hungry or unsatisfied is real but unfounded. It's not about eating less; it's about making informed food choices which give you control over your health, slowly transforming your relationship with food. Implementing this doesn't require drastic changes but rather a few adjustments and a little mindfulness. For example, switching from a large dinner plate to a smaller one can significantly alter your perception of how much food is enough, tricking your brain into feeling satisfied with fewer calories without feeling deprived.

Understanding Serving Sizes

Serving sizes can appear cryptic, often leaving you second-guessing whether you've overstepped the dietary boundaries prescribed for managing diabetes. Every food item has a recommended serving size, which, admittedly, can be less than what emotions might dictate at a famished moment. However, understanding and adhering to these sizes are not meant to strip away the joy of dining but to scaffold your path to a healthier lifestyle.

Start with acquainting yourself with the basics: a serving of meat is the size of a deck of cards; a serving of fruit, about the size of a tennis ball. But beyond memorizing these comparisons, incorporate tools that aid accuracy without becoming a chore. Kitchen scales, measuring cups, and spoons are ambassadors of portion control, ensuring you eat enough to satisfy dietary needs without inadvertently overeating. When you measure out a cup of rice or weigh a piece of fish, you're taking active steps towards maintaining a balanced diet that keeps diabetes management on track.

The Practice of Mindful Eating

Engaging in mindful eating practices transforms the act of eating from a passive to an active process. It's about being present in the moment, acknowledging the flavors, the textures, and the aromas, and respecting your body's signals of hunger and fullness. Eating slowly and savoring each bite can enhance satisfaction from each meal and is instrumental in preventing overeating. This practice is not only a cornerstone in managing weight and diabetes but also in enhancing the overall eating experience, making meals more enjoyable and emotionally fulfilling.

Empowering Through Education

To empower you to make these changes stick, education about nutritional content is indispensable. Knowing the carbohydrate content, the fiber, fat, and sugar level in your foods can aid you in making smarter choices. For instance, opting for fiber-rich foods can impact the rate at which glucose is released into the bloodstream, a paramount aspect for blood sugar management.

A practical approach could involve keeping a food diary initially to track what you eat and how it correlates with your blood sugar readings. This documentation can reveal patterns and help identify which foods spike your blood sugar and which keep it stable, giving you the power to adjust your diet more effectively.

Adjusting With Age

As we age, our metabolism naturally slows down, and our body's needs change. The caloric intake that once suited us in our thirties may become excessive in our fifties and beyond. Adjusting portion sizes to align with a slower metabolism is crucial to avoid weight gain and manage blood sugar levels effectively.

Moreover, as appetite may decrease with age, it becomes even more essential to focus on nutrient-dense foods that provide adequate vitamins, minerals, and other nutrients to keep the body well-fueled and functioning optimally. Prioritizing quality over quantity ensures that every bite contributes to your health without necessarily expanding your waistline.

Implementing Portion Control in Everyday Life

Finally, implementing portion control into your daily routine shouldn't feel like a chore or a compromise but rather an informed choice you make for better health. Integrating small, daily practices such as using smaller plates, measuring servings with standard kitchen tools, and being mindful of the body's cues can gradually lead to profound health improvements.

The goal here is clear—live vibrantly with diabetes, not in spite of it. By mastering the art of portion control and understanding serving sizes, you're not just eating differently; you're embracing a lifestyle that enhances your autonomy over diabetes and enriches your life with every nutritious, carefully measured bite.

5.2 CRAFTING A 28-DAY MEAL PLAN FOR SUCCESS

WEEK 1	breakfast	snack	lunch	snack	dinner
Monday	Berry Blast Smoothie	Acai Bowl with Berries	Grilled Chicken Salad with Avocado	Savory Turmeric Hard-Boiled Eggs	Baked Salmon with Asparagus
Tuesday	Green Power Smoothie	Green Smoothie Bowl with Kiwi	Quinoa and Black Bean Salad	Herb-Infused Turkey Roll-Ups	Chicken Stir-Fry with Broccoli
Wednesday	Tropical Mango Smoothie	Tropical Smoothie Bowl with Coconut	Spinach Salad with Walnuts and Strawberries	Mixed Berry Greek Yogurt Cups	Grilled Tofu with Vegetables
Thursday	Protein-Packed Peanut Butter Smoothie	Protein-Rich Berry Bowl	Greek Salad with Feta and Olives	No-Bake Almond Butter Protein Bars	Beef Tenderloin with Garlic Green Beans
Friday	Avocado Coconut Smoothie	Spiced Pumpkin Smoothie Bowl	Roasted Beet and Goat Cheese Salad	Savory Edamame Hummus Cups	Zesty Lime Shrimp and Avocado Salad
Saturday	Quinoa and Veggie Breakfast Bowl	Roasted Chickpeas	Lentil Soup with Vegetables	Savory Turmeric Hard-Boiled Eggs	Stuffed Bell Peppers with Quinoa
Sunday	Greek Yogurt Parfait with Nuts and Seeds	Spiced Nuts Mix	Chicken and Barley Stew	Herb-Infused Turkey Roll-Ups	Eggplant Parmesan (Low Glycemic)

WEEK 2	breakfast	snack	lunch	snack	dinner
Monday	Steel-Cut Oats with Fresh Berries	Baked Zucchini Chips	Tomato Basil Soup with a Twist	Mixed Berry Greek Yogurt Cups	Roasted Cauliflower Steaks
Tuesday	Chia Pudding with Almond Milk	Kale Chips with Sea Salt	Beef and Vegetable Soup	No-Bake Almond Butter Protein Bars	Zucchini Noodles with Pesto
Wednesday	Savory Millet and Spinach Breakfast Bowl	Crispy Parmesan Edamame Pods	Miso Mushroom Stew	Savory Edamame Hummus Cups	Mediterranean Stuffed Artichokes
Thursday	Berry Blast Smoothie	Apple Slices with Almond Butter	Turkey and Avocado Wrap	Savory Turmeric Hard-Boiled Eggs	Quinoa and Chicken Casserole
Friday	Green Power Smoothie	Carrot Sticks with Hummus	Grilled Veggie Sandwich	Herb-Infused Turkey Roll-Ups	Vegetable and Lentil Curry
Saturday	Tropical Mango Smoothie	Celery with Cottage Cheese	Chicken Caesar Wrap	Mixed Berry Greek Yogurt Cups	Turkey and Sweet Potato Skillet
Sunday	Protein-Packed Peanut Butter Smoothie	Berry and Greek Yogurt Parfait	Tuna Salad Sandwich on Whole Grain Bread	No-Bake Almond Butter Protein Bars	Shrimp and Brown Rice Paella

WEEK 3	breakfast	snack	lunch	snack	dinner
Monday	Avocado Coconut Smoothie	Cucumber Roll-Ups with Avocado Hummus	Mediterranean Tuna and Olive Wrap	Savory Edamame Hummus Cups	Mediterranean Chicken and Quinoa Stew
Tuesday	Quinoa and Veggie Breakfast Bowl	Acai Bowl with Berries	Brown Rice and Veggie Bowl	Savory Turmeric Hard-Boiled Eggs	Whole Wheat Spaghetti with Marinara
Wednesday	Greek Yogurt Parfait with Nuts and Seeds	Green Smoothie Bowl with Kiwi	Barley and Mushroom Bowl	Herb-Infused Turkey Roll-Ups	Brown Rice Pilaf with Herbs
Thursday	Steel-Cut Oats with Fresh Berries	Tropical Smoothie Bowl with Coconut	Farro Salad with Roasted Veggies	Mixed Berry Greek Yogurt Cups	Quinoa Primavera
Friday	Chia Pudding with Almond Milk	Protein-Rich Berry Bowl	Bulgur and Chickpea Bowl	No-Bake Almond Butter Protein Bars	Barley Risotto with Mushrooms
Saturday	Savory Millet and Spinach Breakfast Bowl	Spiced Pumpkin Smoothie Bowl	Quinoa and Pomegranate Delight Bowl	Savory Edamame Hummus Cups	Mediterranean Farro Salad with Grilled Vegetables
Sunday	Berry Blast Smoothie	Roasted Chickpeas	Grilled Chicken Salad with Avocado	Savory Turmeric Hard-Boiled Eggs	Baked Salmon with Asparagus

WEEK 4	breakfast	snack	lunch	snack	dinner
Monday	Green Power Smoothie	Spiced Nuts Mix	Quinoa and Black Bean Salad	Herb-Infused Turkey Roll-Ups	Chicken Stir-Fry with Broccoli
Tuesday	Tropical Mango Smoothie	Baked Zucchini Chips	Spinach Salad with Walnuts and Strawberries	Mixed Berry Greek Yogurt Cups	Grilled Tofu with Vegetables
Wednesday	Protein-Packed Peanut Butter Smoothie	Kale Chips with Sea Salt	Greek Salad with Feta and Olives	No-Bake Almond Butter Protein Bars	Beef Tenderloin with Garlic Green Beans
Thursday	Avocado Coconut Smoothie	Crispy Parmesan Edamame Pods	Roasted Beet and Goat Cheese Salad	Savory Edamame Hummus Cups	Zesty Lime Shrimp and Avocado Salad
Friday	Quinoa and Veggie Breakfast Bowl	Apple Slices with Almond Butter	Lentil Soup with Vegetables	Savory Turmeric Hard-Boiled Eggs	Stuffed Bell Peppers with Quinoa
Saturday	Greek Yogurt Parfait with Nuts and Seeds	Carrot Sticks with Hummus	Chicken and Barley Stew	Herb-Infused Turkey Roll-Ups	Eggplant Parmesan (Low Glycemic)
Sunday	Steel-Cut Oats with Fresh Berries	Celery with Cottage Cheese	Tomato Basil Soup with a Twist	Mixed Berry Greek Yogurt Cups	Roasted Cauliflower Steaks

Welcome to the vibrant world of flexible dining—a concept that encapsulates more than just eating. It's about crafting a meal plan that fits snugly into the jigsaw of your life, irrespective of the pace or style. For those navigating diabetes after 50, adapting a meal strategy that resonates with your lifestyle, cultural preferences, and nutritional needs isn't just a convenience; it's a necessity for sustainable health and happiness.

Living with diabetes does not imply that your food choices should lead you to a culinary dead-end. On the contrary, it opens up a pathway to explore various adjustments and alternatives that promise not merely health but also an indulgence in global palates that tickle your taste buds while keeping your glucose levels balanced.

Customization: The Core of Flexible Meal Planning

The beauty of customizable meal planning is that it acknowledges each individual's unique lifestyle. Whether you are an early riser who loves a hearty breakfast or someone who thrives on small frequent meals throughout the day, your meal plan can and should be adjusted to accommodate these patterns.

Imagine a retiree who now enjoys the leisure of long breakfasts, contrasted with an active professional who may still be working post-50 and needs quick, nutritionally dense breakfast options. Here, customization plays a pivotal role—where the retiree can afford the time to prepare elaborate balanced meals, the professional might benefit from preparing ahead or opting for healthy on-the-go alternatives that fit into a busy morning schedule.

Integrating Personal and Cultural Preferences

Food is deeply intertwined with cultural identity and personal preferences. One aspect of creating a flexible meal plan is ensuring that it respects these elements. For instance, if your diet is primarily plant-based, or if you adhere to cultural dietary restrictions, these factors should seamlessly weave into your diabetic meal plan.

Envision the spices and herbs that paint your cultural canvas—turmeric, basil, oregano—and consider how these could not only flavor your food but also how their health benefits could be utilized. Incorporating such elements adds a layer of personalized touch to your meals, enhancing both their nutritional value and their gastronomic appeal.

Adapting to Social and Family Settings

Social interactions often center around food. A major concern for many managing diabetes is how to balance social dining without navigating a minefield of unsuitable food choices. Flexibility in your meal plan means having strategies up your sleeve for such situations.

Preparing ahead of events by ensuring the meals leading up to social gatherings are particularly balanced, or having a repertoire of diabetes-friendly dishes that can be shared with friends and family can alleviate stress. Moreover, educating close ones about your dietary considerations can not only increase your comfort but also broaden the communal support in your journey towards health.

Harnessing the Power of Technology

In this digital age, dietary management for diabetes can be streamlined with apps and tools designed to track your eating habits, forecast your needs, and even generate meal suggestions tailored to your medical and personal preferences. These tools can be especially useful for varying daily schedules, shifting the brunt of meal planning from daunting to doable.

Leverage technology to remind you of meal times, keep track of carbohydrate intake, and even provide shopping lists that align with your meal plans. These digital assistants ensure that no matter your lifestyle pace or changes, your meal strategy adapts accordingly.

Responding to Changes in Health Status

As we age, our health status may change, and with it, our nutritional needs can also shift. Flexibility in meal planning means these changes are taken into account dynamically. Whether dealing with weight management issues, adjusting for increased physical activity, or responding to changes in medication—your meal plan can evolve.

An approach that marries the principles of sound nutrition with the specifics of your health metrics can ensure that your meal plan is not just a static regimen but a responsive, evolving framework. Regular consultations with nutrition experts and medical practitioners can guide these adjustments, ensuring your meal plan remains as dynamic as your life.

Conclusion

Your journey with diabetes is deeply personal, and your meal plan should reflect this uniqueness. Embracing flexibility doesn't just cater to your tastes and lifestyle; it respects the depth and breadth of your life's experiences and plans. Each meal then becomes not just a routine you have to follow, but a choice you delight in, one that fits seamlessly into the tapestry of your everyday life. This way, managing diabetes becomes not just about health—it is about living your best life, every single day.

PART III: DELICIOUS AND HEALTHY RECIPES

CHAPTER 6: BREAKFAST RECIPES

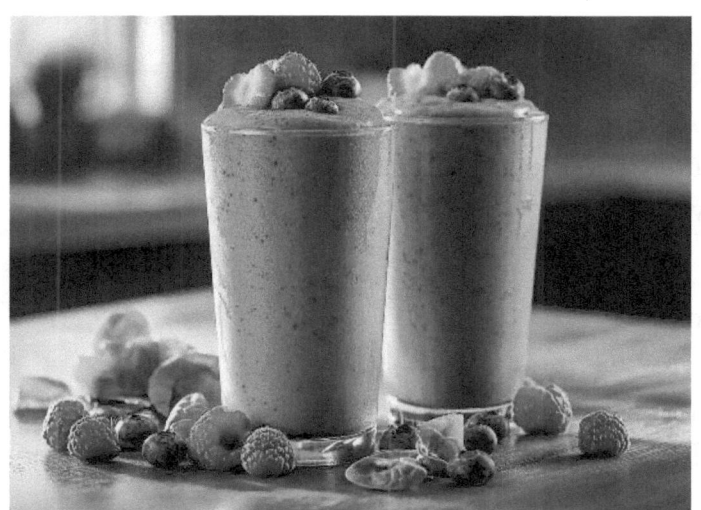

Ah, breakfast! Often hailed as the most important meal of the day, its significance skyrockets when you're managing diabetes post-50. It's not just about quelling the morning hunger or sipping that invigorating cup of coffee. For you, it's about kickstarting your day with stability, nurturing your body in a way that keeps your blood sugars balanced and your energy levels adequately high. Imagine waking up to a meal that not only tastes delightful but also fortifies your health, aligns with your body's needs, and sets a positive tone for the hours to come. Breakfast, in the world of diabetes management, transcends mere eating; it's a thoughtful ritual that embraces nourishment and conscious choices.

Yet, I know the concerns that might be brewing in your mind. Will these recipes be tasty? Are they going to be yet another bland iteration of diabetic stereotypes? Let me put those fears to rest. Each recipe crafted and curated in this chapter ensures that flavor and health are not mutually exclusive. From the aromatic spices that will fill your morning kitchen to the fresh, vibrant colors of your plate, each dish is designed to appeal not only to your palette but also to your visual senses.

As we step through this chapter, every recipe will reveal the secrets of low glycemic ingredients that don't spike your blood sugar, combined in ways that are innovative and sometimes, delightfully surprising. Think cinnamon-infused oatmeal, but with a twist that includes a sprinkle of nutrient-rich chia seeds, or perhaps a savory muffin that packs both taste and protein without the carb overload.

I invite you to treat these breakfast recipes not just as a meal, but as your first victory of the day — a testament to your resolve to manage diabetes with joy and not just with discipline. It's about making that silver lining in your cloud very real, every morning. Remember, in your journey through diabetes management after 50, how you start your day often determines how well you live it. So, let's start it right — together.

6.1. LOW GLYCEMIC SMOOTHIES

BERRY BLAST SMOOTHIE

Preparation Time: 5 min - **Cooking Time:** none - **Servings:** 2 Serv.
Glycemic Index: Low(~35)
Ingredients:
- 1 C. mixed berries (blueberries, strawberries, raspberries), frozen

- 1 C. spinach, fresh
- 1 C. Greek yogurt, low-fat
- 1 Tbsp honey, raw
- 1 tsp vanilla extract
- 1 C. almond milk, unsweetened

Directions:

1. Combine all ingredients in a high-speed blender and blend until smooth
2. Pour into two glasses and serve immediately

Tips:
- Add a scoop of protein powder for an extra boost
- Use ice if using fresh berries for a chilled version
- Blend for an extra minute for a smoother texture

Nutritional Values: Calories: 150, Fat: 2g, Carbs: 25g, Protein: 8g, Sugar: 18g, Sodium: 60 mg, Potassium: 350 mg, Cholesterol: 5 mg

GREEN POWER SMOOTHIE

Preparation Time: 7 min - **Cooking Time:** none - **Servings:** 1
Glycemic Index: Low(~40)
Ingredients:
- 1 C. kale, fresh, de-stemmed
- ½ avocado, peeled and pitted
- 1 small banana, sliced
- 1 Tbsp chia seeds
- 1 Tbsp almond butter
- 1½ C. coconut water
- 1 tsp spirulina powder

Directions:

1. Place kale, avocado, banana, almond butter, chia seeds, and spirulina in a blender
2. Add coconut water and blend until smooth
3. Serve chilled in a tall glass

Tips:
- Opt for organic kale to reduce pesticide intake
- Add a bit of lemon juice to enhance freshness and prolong shelf life

Nutritional Values: Calories: 320, Fat: 15g, Carbs: 44g, Protein: 8g, Sugar: 20g, Sodium: 150 mg, Potassium: 890 mg, Cholesterol: 0 mg

TROPICAL MANGO SMOOTHIE

Preparation Time: 6 min - **Cooking Time:** none - **Servings:** 2
Glycemic Index: Low(~45)

Ingredients:

- 1 C. mango, frozen
- ½ C. pineapple, chopped
- 1 C. Greek yogurt, low-fat
- 1 tsp lime zest
- ½ tsp turmeric, ground
- 1 C. coconut milk, light

Directions:

1. Blend mango, pineapple, Greek yogurt, lime zest, and turmeric in a blender until creamy
2. Gradually add coconut milk and blend until smooth
3. Serve immediately in chilled glasses

Tips:

- Experiment with a pinch of cayenne pepper for a spicy kick
- Substitute pineapple with papaya for different flavors

Nutritional Values: Calories: 215, Fat: 5g, Carbs: 35g, Protein: 8g, Sugar: 28g, Sodium: 45 mg, Potassium: 500 mg, Cholesterol: 10 mg

PROTEIN-PACKED PEANUT BUTTER SMOOTHIE

Preparation Time: 8 min - **Cooking Time:** none - **Servings:** 2
Glycemic Index: Low(~40)

Ingredients:

- 2 Tbsp peanut butter, natural, unsweetened
- 1 small banana, frozen
- 1 C. Greek yogurt, low-fat
- 1 Tbsp flaxseed, ground
- 1 C. soy milk, unsweetened
- 1 tsp cinnamon, ground

Directions:

1. Add peanut butter, banana, Greek yogurt, ground flaxseed, and cinnamon to a blender
2. Pour in soy milk
3. Blend until the mixture is smooth and creamy
4. Serve in two glasses

Tips:

- Use almond butter if allergic to peanuts
- Sprinkle a dash of nutmeg for added spice
- Freeze the banana in slices for easier blending

Nutritional Values: Calories: 310, Fat: 16g, Carbs: 30g, Protein: 15g, Sugar: 18g, Sodium: 95 mg, Potassium: 650 mg, Cholesterol: 8 mg

Preparation Time: 5 min - **Cooking Time:** none - **Servings:** 1

Glycemic Index: Low(~35)

Ingredients:

- 1 ripe avocado, peeled and pitted
- 1 C. coconut milk, unsweetened
- 1 Tbsp chia seeds
- ½ tsp vanilla extract
- 1 Tbsp lime juice
- 2 tsp stevia
- ½ C. ice cubes

Directions:

1. Combine avocado, coconut milk, chia seeds, vanilla extract, lime juice, stevia, and ice cubes in a blender and blend until smooth
2. Taste and adjust sweetness or acidity, depending on your preference
3. Serve chilled in a tall glass

Tips:

- Consider adding a pinch of matcha powder for an antioxidant boost and a vibrant color
- Top with a sprinkling of unsweetened shredded coconut for extra texture and flavor
- For a protein boost, blend in a scoop of your preferred plant-based protein powder

Nutritional Values: Calories: 345, Fat: 29g, Carbs: 21g, Protein: 4g, Sugar: 3g, Sodium: 15 mg, Potassium: 708 mg, Cholesterol: 0 mg

6.2. HEARTY BREAKFAST BOWLS

QUINOA AND VEGGIE BREAKFAST BOWL

Preparation Time: 15 min - **Cooking Time:** 20 min - **Servings:** 2

Glycemic Index: Low(~50)

Ingredients:

- ½ C. quinoa, rinsed
- 1 C. water
- ½ small zucchini, diced
- ½ red bell pepper, chopped
- ¼ C. red onion, finely chopped
- 1 clove garlic, minced
- 1 Tbsp olive oil
- 2 eggs, poached or fried
- Salt and pepper to taste
- ¼ tsp paprika

Directions:

1. Add quinoa and water to a saucepan, bring to boil, then cover and simmer for 15 min until water is absorbed
2. In a skillet, heat olive oil over medium heat; sauté zucchini, bell pepper, onion, and garlic until soft
3. Mix cooked vegetables with quinoa, season with paprika, salt, and pepper
4. Serve in bowls topped with poached or fried eggs

Tips:

- Add a squeeze of fresh lemon juice for zest
- Top with chopped fresh herbs like parsley or cilantro for enhanced flavor

Nutritional Values: Calories: 350, Fat: 15g, Carbs: 40g, Protein: 14g, Sugar: 4g, Sodium: 150 mg, Potassium: 530 mg, Cholesterol: 186 mg

GREEK YOGURT PARFAIT WITH NUTS AND SEEDS

Preparation Time: 5 min - **Cooking Time:** none - **Servings:** 1
Glycemic Index: Low(~35)
Ingredients:

- 1 C. Greek yogurt, low-fat
- 2 Tbsp mixed nuts (almonds, walnuts), chopped
- 1 Tbsp sunflower seeds
- 1 Tbsp pumpkin seeds
- ½ C. mixed berries (strawberries, blueberries)
- 1 tsp honey, optional

Directions:

1. Arrange a layer of Greek yogurt at the bottom of a glass
2. Add a layer of mixed nuts and seeds
3. Add a layer of mixed berries
4. Repeat the layering if desired
5. Drizzle with honey if using

Tips:

- Substitute honey with a light drizzle of agave syrup for a lower GI option
- Use organic seeds and nuts for better nutrient retention

Nutritional Values: Calories: 310, Fat: 18g, Carbs: 24g, Protein: 20g, Sugar: 12g, Sodium: 85 mg, Potassium: 345 mg, Cholesterol: 10 mg

STEEL-CUT OATS WITH FRESH BERRIES

Preparation Time: 5 min - **Cooking Time:** 30 min - **Servings:** 2
Glycemic Index: Low(~40)

Ingredients:

- ¼ C. steel-cut oats
- 1¼ C. water
- Pinch of salt
- ½ C. fresh strawberries, sliced
- ½ C. fresh blueberries
- 1 Tbsp honey, optional
- 1 tsp ground cinnamon

Directions:

1. Combine steel-cut oats, water, and a pinch of salt in a medium saucepan and bring to a boil
2. Reduce heat to low and simmer, stirring occasionally, for 25-30 min until oats are tender
3. Serve hot topped with sliced strawberries, blueberries, cinnamon, and a drizzle of honey if desired

Tips:

- Sweeten with a drizzle of stevia or monk fruit syrup for an even lower GI
- Keep a watchful eye on oats to prevent sticking and burning

Nutritional Values: Calories: 185, Fat: 2g, Carbs: 38g, Protein: 6g, Sugar: 10g, Sodium: 60 mg, Potassium: 169 mg, Cholesterol: 0 mg

CHIA PUDDING WITH ALMOND MILK

Preparation Time: 10 min - **Cooking Time:** none - **Servings:** 2
Glycemic Index: Low(~35)
Ingredients:

- 2 Tbsp chia seeds
- 1 C. almond milk, unsweetened
- ½ tsp vanilla extract
- 1 Tbsp maple syrup, optional
- ½ C. fresh mango, diced
- 2 Tbsp coconut flakes, unsweetened

Directions:

1. Combine chia seeds, almond milk, vanilla extract, and maple syrup in a bowl; stir well
2. Cover and refrigerate for at least 2 hrs or overnight until pudding is thickened
3. Serve topped with diced mango and coconut flakes

Tips:

- Experiment with different fruits such as kiwi or ripe pears for variety
- Opt for organic almond milk for a cleaner ingredient profile

Nutritional Values: Calories: 215, Fat: 9g, Carbs: 30g, Protein: 5g, Sugar: 15g, Sodium: 95 mg, Potassium: 222 mg, Cholesterol: 0 mg

Preparation Time: 15 min - **Cooking Time:** 20 min - **Servings:** 2

Glycemic Index: Low(~50)

Ingredients:

- ½ C. millet, dry
- 1½ C. water
- 1 pinch sea salt
- 2 C. fresh spinach, chopped
- 2 large eggs
- 1 tsp olive oil
- ¼ C. feta cheese, crumbled
- 1 tsp turmeric
- ½ tsp black pepper

Directions:

1. Rinse millet thoroughly and combine with water and sea salt in a medium saucepan
2. Bring to a boil, then reduce heat to low, cover, and simmer for 18 min or until water is absorbed
3. In a separate pan, heat olive oil over medium, add spinach, and sauté until wilted
4. Crack eggs into the pan with spinach, sprinkle turmeric and pepper, and cook until eggs are set
5. Fluff cooked millet with a fork, then divide between two bowls, topping each with spinach and an egg, and sprinkle with feta cheese

Tips:

- Opt for organic spinach to minimize pesticide intake
- Add a pinch of cayenne for a spicy kick
- Serve with a slice of whole-grain bread for extra fiber

Nutritional Values: Calories: 320, Fat: 15g, Carbs: 36g, Protein: 14g, Sugar: 2g, Sodium: 370 mg, Potassium: 510 mg, Cholesterol: 186 mg

6.3. EGG-BASED DISHES

SPINACH AND FETA OMELET

Preparation Time: 15 min - **Cooking Time:** 10 min - **Servings:** 1

Glycemic Index: Low(~30)

Ingredients:

- 2 large eggs
- 1 cup spinach, fresh, chopped
- 2 Tbsp feta cheese, crumbled
- 1 Tbsp olive oil

- ¼ tsp black pepper, freshly ground
- 1 clove garlic, minced

Directions:

1. Whisk eggs with black pepper and set aside
2. Heat olive oil in a skillet over medium heat
3. Saute garlic until fragrant, about 1 min
4. Add spinach and cook until wilted, about 3 min
5. Pour eggs over spinach, sprinkle feta on top, and cook until eggs are set, about 6 min, folding omelet in half during the last minute of cooking

Tips:

- Use organic spinach for better flavor and nutrient content
- Add a dash of nutmeg to the eggs for enhanced depth of flavor
- Serve with a slice of whole grain toast for added fiber

Nutritional Values: Calories: 290, Fat: 23g, Carbs: 4g, Protein: 19g, Sugar: 2g, Sodium: 410 mg, Potassium: 240 mg, Cholesterol: 370 mg

AVOCADO AND TOMATO SCRAMBLE

Preparation Time: 10 min - **Cooking Time:** 8 min - **Servings:** 1
Glycemic Index: Low(~35)
Ingredients:

- 2 large eggs
- ½ avocado, diced
- ½ cup cherry tomatoes, halved
- 1 Tbsp chives, chopped
- 1 tsp olive oil
- Salt and pepper to taste

Directions:

1. Beat the eggs with salt and pepper in a bowl
2. Heat olive oil in a pan over medium heat
3. Add tomatoes and cook until they are soft, about 4 min
4. Add eggs and scramble gently
5. Halfway through, add diced avocado and chives, continue cooking until eggs are fully set

Tips:

- Opt for ripe avocados for creaminess
- Serve immediately to maintain the freshness of the avocado
- A sprinkle of red pepper flakes can add a nice kick

Nutritional Values: Calories: 320, Fat: 25g, Carbs: 9g, Protein: 13g, Sugar: 2g, Sodium: 210 mg, Potassium: 560 mg, Cholesterol: 372 mg

Preparation Time: 15 min - **Cooking Time:** 20 min - **Servings:** 6

Glycemic Index: Low(~40)

Ingredients:

- 6 large eggs
- 1 cup bell peppers, diced
- 1 cup broccoli florets, finely chopped
- ½ cup onions, finely diced
- ¼ cup milk, low-fat
- ½ cup cheddar cheese, shredded
- Salt and pepper to taste
- Cooking spray

Directions:

1. Preheat oven to 375°F (190°C)
2. Whisk eggs, milk, salt, and pepper together in a large bowl
3. Stir in bell peppers, broccoli, onions, and cheese
4. Coat a muffin tin with cooking spray and pour the egg mixture into the muffin cups
5. Bake for 20 min until muffins are set

Tips:

- Fill muffin cups only three-quarters full to prevent overflow as they bake
- Use any combination of veggies like spinach or zucchini for variety
- These muffins can be stored in the refrigerator for quick breakfast options throughout the week

Nutritional Values: Calories: 150, Fat: 10g, Carbs: 6g, Protein: 9g, Sugar: 3g, Sodium: 220 mg, Potassium: 180 mg, Cholesterol: 185 mg

POACHED EGGS ON WHOLE GRAIN TOAST

Preparation Time: 10 min - **Cooking Time:** 4 min - **Servings:** 1

Glycemic Index: Low(~35)

Ingredients:

- 2 large eggs
- 2 slices whole grain bread, toasted
- 1 tsp vinegar
- Salt and pepper to taste
- 1 Tbsp parsley, chopped

Directions:

1. Bring a pot of water to a light simmer and add vinegar
2. Crack eggs into separate cups then gently slide into simmering water
3. Poach eggs for about 4 min until the whites are set but yolks remain runny

4. Remove with a slotted spoon and drain on kitchen paper
5. Serve on toasted whole grain bread, season with salt and pepper, garnish with parsley

Tips:
- Adding vinegar to the poaching water helps the egg whites to coagulate more effectively
- Use freshly ground black pepper for a robust flavor
- Garnish with other fresh herbs like chives or dill if desired

Nutritional Values: Calories: 270, Fat: 12g, Carbs: 28g, Protein: 16g, Sugar: 4g, Sodium: 410 mg, Potassium: 220 mg, Cholesterol: 370 mg

SHAKSHUKA WITH GOAT CHEESE

Preparation Time: 15 min - **Cooking Time:** 25 min - **Servings:** 4

Glycemic Index: Low(~40)

Ingredients:
- 2 Tbsp olive oil
- 1 medium onion, diced
- 1 red bell pepper, diced
- 2 cloves garlic, minced
- 1 tsp cumin, ground
- 1 tsp paprika, smoked
- ¼ tsp chili powder
- 1 can (14 oz.) tomatoes, diced
- 6 large eggs
- 2 oz. goat cheese, crumbled
- 2 Tbsp parsley, fresh, chopped
- Salt to taste
- Black pepper to taste

Directions:

1. Heat olive oil in a large skillet over medium heat
2. Add onion and bell pepper, sauté until softened
3. Stir in garlic, cumin, paprika, and chili powder, cook for 1 min
4. Pour in diced tomatoes and season with salt and pepper, simmer for 10 min
5. Crack eggs into the sauce, spacing evenly
6. Cover and cook until eggs are set
7. Crumble goat cheese and sprinkle parsley over the top before serving

Tips:
- Use fresh herbs to enhance flavor
- Serve with a slice of whole-grain bread to complete the meal

Nutritional Values: Calories: 225, Fat: 15g, Carbs: 10g, Protein: 13g, Sugar: 6g, Sodium: 320 mg, Potassium: 364 mg, Cholesterol: 210 mg

ALMOND FLOUR PANCAKES

Preparation Time: 15 min - **Cooking Time:** 10 min - **Servings:** 4

Glycemic Index: Low(~30)

Ingredients:

- 2 cups almond flour
- 1 tsp baking powder
- 1/4 tsp salt
- 1/4 tsp cinnamon, ground
- 2 eggs, large
- 1/2 cup almond milk, unsweetened
- 1 Tbsp coconut oil, melted
- 1 tsp vanilla extract

Directions:

1. Mix almond flour, baking powder, salt, and cinnamon in one bowl
2. Whisk eggs, almond milk, melted coconut oil, and vanilla extract in another bowl
3. Combine wet and dry ingredients, stir until smooth
4. Heat a non-stick griddle over medium heat and pour 1/4 cup batter for each pancake
5. Cook until bubbles form on the surface, then flip and cook until golden on both sides

Tips:

- Opt for monk fruit sweetener to add sweetness without affecting GI
- Serve with a dollop of Greek yogurt for added protein

Nutritional Values: Calories: 315, Fat: 25g, Carbs: 12g, Protein: 13g, Sugar: 1g, Sodium: 300 mg, Potassium: 150 mg, Cholesterol: 93 mg

WHOLE WHEAT WAFFLES WITH FRESH FRUIT

Preparation Time: 10 min - **Cooking Time:** 5 min - **Servings:** 3

Glycemic Index: Medium(~58)

Ingredients:

- 1 1/2 cups whole wheat flour
- 1 Tbsp baking powder
- 1/2 tsp salt
- 2 Tbsp sugar substitute
- 1 egg, large
- 1 cup low-fat milk
- 1/4 cup vegetable oil
- 1 tsp vanilla extract
- 1 cup mixed berries (strawberries, blueberries, raspberries), fresh

Directions:

1. Combine whole wheat flour, baking powder, salt, and sugar substitute in a bowl
2. In another bowl, beat the egg with low-fat milk, vegetable oil, and vanilla extract
3. Mix wet ingredients into dry until smooth
4. Heat waffle iron and pour batter, cook until crisp
5. Serve topped with fresh mixed berries

Tips:
- Experiment with different berries for varied flavor and antioxidant benefits
- Use organic extracts for natural flavoring

Nutritional Values: Calories: 280, Fat: 11g, Carbs: 39g, Protein: 8g, Sugar: 10g, Sodium: 450 mg, Potassium: 222 mg, Cholesterol: 54 mg

FLAXSEED PANCAKES WITH BLUEBERRIES

Preparation Time: 20 min - **Cooking Time:** 15 min - **Servings:** 2

Glycemic Index: Low(~50)

Ingredients:
- 1 cup whole wheat flour
- 2 Tbsp ground flaxseed
- 1 tsp baking powder
- 1/2 tsp cinnamon, ground
- 2 Tbsp maple syrup, sugar-free
- 1 cup low-fat buttermilk
- 1 egg
- 1/2 cup blueberries, fresh
- 1 Tbsp coconut oil, for griddle

Directions:

1. Sift together whole wheat flour, ground flaxseed, baking powder, and cinnamon
2. Whisk in low-fat buttermilk, egg, and sugar-free maple syrup until smooth
3. Heat a griddle to medium heat and brush with coconut oil
4. Pour batter and sprinkle blueberries on top, flip when bubbles form and cook til done

Tips:
- Enhance flavor by adding a pinch of nutmeg or cardamom to the batter
- Serve with a drizzle of warmed, sugar-free maple syrup

Nutritional Values: Calories: 290, Fat: 9g, Carbs: 44g, Protein: 11g, Sugar: 12g, Sodium: 380 mg, Potassium: 200 mg, Cholesterol: 95 mg

CINNAMON-SPICED OAT WAFFLES

Preparation Time: 15 min - **Cooking Time:** 10 min - **Servings:** 3

Glycemic Index: Low(~40)

Ingredients:

- 1 1/2 cups rolled oats
- 1/2 cup almond flour
- 1 Tbsp ground cinnamon
- 2 tsp baking powder
- 1/4 tsp salt
- 1 1/2 cups almond milk, unsweetened
- 2 eggs
- 1 Tbsp olive oil
- 2 tsp vanilla extract

Directions:

1. Grind rolled oats into flour using a food processor
2. Mix oat flour, almond flour, cinnamon, baking powder, and salt in a bowl
3. In a separate bowl, whisk together unsweetened almond milk, eggs, olive oil, and vanilla
4. Combine wet and dry ingredients until smooth
5. Heat waffle iron and cook batter until golden and crispy

Tips:

- Add a few drops of vanilla stevia for extra sweetness without the sugar
- Top with a dash of cinnamon right before serving for a fresher spice hit

Nutritional Values: Calories: 255, Fat: 15g, Carbs: 27g, Protein: 9g, Sugar: 1g, Sodium: 350 mg, Potassium: 235 mg, Cholesterol: 124 mg

BUCKWHEAT AND ZUCCHINI PANCAKES

Preparation Time: 15 min - **Cooking Time:** 10 min - **Servings:** 4

Glycemic Index: Low(~50)

Ingredients:

- 1 C. buckwheat flour
- 1 small zucchini, grated
- 2 eggs, large
- 1 C. almond milk, unsweetened
- 1 tsp baking powder
- ½ tsp salt
- 1 tsp olive oil for cooking
- 1 Tbsp flaxseed meal

Directions:

1. Whisk eggs and almond milk in a mixing bowl until uniform
2. Stir in grated zucchini
3. In another bowl, combine buckwheat flour, baking powder, salt, and flaxseed meal
4. Gradually fold the dry ingredients into the wet mixture until well combined
5. Heat olive oil in a non-stick skillet over medium heat
6. Pour batter to form pancakes, cook until bubbles form on the top, then flip to cook the other side until golden

Tips:
- For extra fluffiness, let the batter rest for 5-10 minutes before cooking
- Serve with a dollop of Greek yogurt or sugar-free apple sauce for added moisture without the sugar spike

Nutritional Values: Calories: 175, Fat: 5g, Carbs: 27g, Protein: 8g, Sugar: 2g, Sodium: 300 mg, Potassium: 250 mg, Cholesterol: 95 mg

CHAPTER 7: LUNCH RECIPES

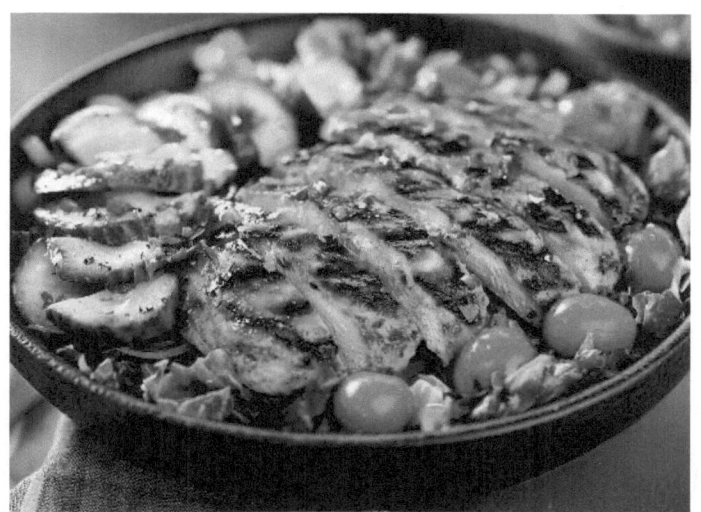

Ah, the midday meal! Lunch often holds the balance of our daily mood and energy, something even more true for those managing diabetes past the age of fifty. As we delve into the delicious world of lunch recipes tailored for a low glycemic lifestyle, think of it not just as a list of meals but as an invitation to an enjoyable, healthful midday break that the whole family can look forward to. Imagine yourself in your kitchen where the sun peeks through the blinds, casting a warm glow over a countertop lined with vibrant vegetables and wholesome proteins. This chapter is designed to transform that everyday picture into a reality — without the stress often associated with 'diet food'. Each recipe here is more than its components. It's a bridge to maintaining your blood sugar levels, sure; but also to revitalizing your afternoons, sustaining your energy till dinner, and keeping you connected to your culinary passions and sharing them with others.

We will wander through a range of delicious, easy-to-prepare dishes—from rejuvenating salads that tickle your taste buds with tangy dressings to hearty, comforting soups that wrap you like a warm hug. How about a savory, grilled chicken with a spice rub that whispers hints of the Mediterranean, or a crisp, colorful salad bursting with flavors and textures that dance in your mouth? Yes, these lunches do more than just fit your diabetic diet; they excite your palate and respect your time constraints.

Moreover, these recipes ensure that you step out of the usual sandwich and chips routine, introducing ingredients that maybe you've passed by during grocery trips. With every bite, you're not just nourishing your body; you're also making strides in your journey of diabetic management through enjoyable and sustaining meals.

So, let's turn the page on mundane, and embrace a midday meal that continues your path of health and pleasure, proving that a diabetic diet after fifty can indeed be as flavorful and varied as any gourmet experience. Here's to lunches that look good, taste marvelous, and work hard for your health—just like you.

7.1. FRESH AND FILLING SALADS

GRILLED CHICKEN SALAD WITH AVOCADO

Preparation Time: 15 min - **Cooking Time:** 10 min - **Servings:** 4
Glycemic Index: Low(~45)
Ingredients:
- 2 chicken breasts, skinless and boneless

- 1 avocado, sliced
- 1 romaine lettuce head, chopped
- 1 cucumber, diced
- 10 cherry tomatoes, halved
- 1 red onion, thinly sliced
- 2 Tbsp olive oil
- 1 Tbsp balsamic vinegar
- 1 lemon, juiced
- Salt and pepper to taste

Directions:

1. Season chicken breasts with salt and pepper
2. Grill chicken over medium heat until cooked through, about 5 min on each side
3. Let chicken rest for 5 min, then slice
4. In a large salad bowl, combine lettuce, cucumber, cherry tomatoes, and red onion
5. Add grilled chicken slices and avocado on top
6. In a small bowl, whisk together olive oil, balsamic vinegar, and lemon juice
7. Drizzle dressing over salad and toss gently

Tips:
- Use freshly squeezed lemon juice for the dressing for a fresher taste
- For a smokier flavor, grill the chicken over charcoal
- Add a pinch of chili flakes to the dressing for a slight kick

Nutritional Values: Calories: 290, Fat: 15g, Carbs: 12g, Protein: 25g, Sugar: 3g, Sodium: 120 mg, Potassium: 790 mg, Cholesterol: 60 mg

QUINOA AND BLACK BEAN SALAD

Preparation Time: 20 min - **Cooking Time:** 15 min - **Servings:** 4
Glycemic Index: Low(~35)

Ingredients:
- 1 C. quinoa
- 1 C. black beans, cooked and drained
- 1 red bell pepper, diced
- 1/4 C. fresh cilantro, chopped
- 1/4 C. green onions, chopped
- 1/4 tsp cumin
- Juice of 2 limes
- 2 Tbsp extra-virgin olive oil
- Salt and pepper to taste

Directions:

1. Rinse quinoa under cold water until the water runs clear

2. Cook quinoa in boiling water for 15 min, then fluff with a fork and cool
3. In a large bowl, mix together cooled quinoa, black beans, red bell pepper, cilantro, and green onions
4. In a small bowl whisk together lime juice, olive oil, cumin, salt, and pepper to create the dressing
5. Pour dressing over salad and mix well

Tips:
- Serve chilled or at room temperature for best flavor
- Adjust lime juice and olive oil quantities based on personal taste preference

Nutritional Values: Calories: 210, Fat: 7g, Carbs: 30g, Protein: 8g, Sugar: 1g, Sodium: 30 mg, Potassium: 480 mg, Cholesterol: 0 mg

SPINACH SALAD WITH WALNUTS AND STRAWBERRIES

Preparation Time: 10 min - **Cooking Time:** none - **Servings:** 4
Glycemic Index: Low(~40)
Ingredients:
- 4 C. fresh spinach leaves
- 1 C. strawberries, sliced
- 1/2 C. walnuts, chopped
- 1/4 C. goat cheese, crumbled
- 2 Tbsp balsamic vinaigrette
- 1 Tbsp honey
- Salt and pepper to taste

Directions:

1. In a large salad bowl, combine spinach, strawberries, and walnuts
2. Crumble goat cheese over the top
3. In a small bowl, whisk together balsamic vinaigrette, honey, salt, and pepper
4. Drizzle the dressing over the salad and toss gently to combine

Tips:
- Opt for organic strawberries for the best taste and health benefits
- Toast walnuts before adding to the salad for enhanced flavor and crunch

Nutritional Values: Calories: 250, Fat: 20g, Carbs: 16g, Protein: 6g, Sugar: 10g, Sodium: 170 mg, Potassium: 350 mg, Cholesterol: 15 mg

GREEK SALAD WITH FETA AND OLIVES

Preparation Time: 10 min - **Cooking Time:** none - **Servings:** 4
Glycemic Index: Low(~40)
Ingredients:
- 1 romaine lettuce head, chopped

- 1 C. cherry tomatoes, halved
- 1 cucumber, sliced
- 1/2 C. Kalamata olives, pitted
- 1/2 red onion, thinly sliced
- 200 g feta cheese, crumbled
- 3 Tbsp olive oil
- 1 Tbsp red wine vinegar
- 1 tsp dried oregano
- Salt and pepper to taste

Directions:

1. In a large salad bowl, combine lettuce, tomatoes, cucumber, olives, and onion
2. Sprinkle feta cheese on top
3. In a small bowl, mix together olive oil, red wine vinegar, oregano, salt, and pepper to create the dressing
4. Pour dressing over the salad and toss to coat thoroughly

Tips:
- For a creamier texture, use a block of feta and crumble it yourself
- Garnish with fresh parsley for added color and flavor

Nutritional Values: Calories: 250, Fat: 21g, Carbs: 8g, Protein: 7g, Sugar: 4g, Sodium: 620 mg, Potassium: 240 mg, Cholesterol: 25 mg

ROASTED BEET AND GOAT CHEESE SALAD

Preparation Time: 15 min - **Cooking Time:** 25 min - **Servings:** 4

Glycemic Index: Low(~40)

Ingredients:
- 3 medium beets, scrubbed and trimmed
- 2 Tbsp olive oil
- 1 tsp sea salt
- 1/2 tsp freshly ground black pepper
- 4 cups arugula leaves
- 1/2 cup crumbled goat cheese
- 1/4 cup walnuts, toasted and chopped
- 2 Tbsp balsamic vinegar reduction

Directions:

1. Preheat oven to 400°F (200°C)
2. Toss beets with olive oil, salt, and pepper and wrap individually in foil
3. Roast in the oven until tender, about 25 min
4. Once cool, peel and dice beets
5. Combine arugula, diced beets, goat cheese, and walnuts in a salad bowl

6. Drizzle with balsamic reduction just before serving

Tips:
- Add a sprinkle of fresh herbs like parsley or mint for a fresh touch
- Substitute walnuts with pecans if preferred for a different nutty flavor

Nutritional Values: Calories: 210, Fat: 15g, Carbs: 13g, Protein: 6g, Sugar: 8g, Sodium: 400 mg, Potassium: 440 mg, Cholesterol: 13 mg

7.2. SAVORY SOUPS AND STEWS

LENTIL SOUP WITH VEGETABLES

Preparation Time: 15 min - **Cooking Time:** 45 min - **Servings:** 4
Glycemic Index: Low(~40)
Ingredients:
- 1 cup lentils, rinsed
- 1 Tbsp olive oil
- 1 medium onion, chopped
- 2 garlic cloves, minced
- 2 carrots, diced
- 2 celery stalks, diced
- 1 bay leaf
- 6 cups vegetable broth, low sodium
- 1 tsp dried thyme
- ½ tsp black pepper, freshly ground
- 1 cup spinach, chopped
- 2 Tbsp parsley, fresh, chopped

Directions:

1. Heat the olive oil in a large pot over medium heat
2. Sauté the onion and garlic until translucent, about 5 minutes
3. Add carrots and celery, continue to cook for another 5 minutes
4. Stir in lentils, bay leaf, thyme, black pepper, and vegetable broth
5. Bring to a boil, reduce heat to low, and simmer covered for 35 minutes or until lentils are tender
6. Add spinach and cook for another 5 minutes
7. Remove bay leaf and garnish with fresh parsley before serving

Tips:
- Consider drizzling a teaspoon of lemon juice for added zest just before serving
- Use freshly ground black pepper for best flavor
- For a heartier texture, add a spoonful of cooked quinoa into each bowl before serving

Nutritional Values: Calories: 230, Fat: 3g, Carbs: 35g, Protein: 12g, Sugar: 5g, Sodium: 300 mg, Potassium: 470 mg, Cholesterol: 0 mg

CHICKEN AND BARLEY STEW

Preparation Time: 20 min - **Cooking Time:** 1 hr - **Servings:** 4

Glycemic Index: Low(~50)

Ingredients:

- 2 chicken breasts, boneless and skinless, cubed
- 1 Tbsp olive oil
- 1 onion, chopped
- 2 garlic cloves, minced
- 3 carrots, sliced
- 2 celery stalks, sliced
- ½ cup pearled barley
- 6 cups chicken broth, low sodium
- 1 tsp dried rosemary
- ½ tsp black pepper, freshly ground
- 1 cup kale, stems removed and chopped

Directions:

1. Heat olive oil in a large pot over medium heat
2. Cook chicken cubes until lightly browned, about 5 minutes, set aside
3. In the same pot, add onion and garlic, sauté until soft, about 5 minutes
4. Add carrots, celery, barley, chicken, chicken broth, rosemary, and black pepper
5. Bring to a boil, then reduce heat to a simmer, cover, and cook for about 50 minutes, or until barley is tender
6. Stir in kale during the last 10 minutes of cooking

Tips:

- Roast garlic before adding for a more caramelized flavor
- Switch kale with swiss chard for a different nutrient profile
- Add a splash of white wine while cooking chicken for extra flavor

Nutritional Values: Calories: 295, Fat: 6g, Carbs: 35g, Protein: 22g, Sugar: 5g, Sodium: 410 mg, Potassium: 650 mg, Cholesterol: 55 mg

TOMATO BASIL SOUP WITH A TWIST

Preparation Time: 10 min - **Cooking Time:** 30 min - **Servings:** 4

Glycemic Index: Low(~38)

Ingredients:

- 2 cups tomatoes, chopped
- 1 onion, diced

- 2 garlic cloves, minced
- 1 Tbsp olive oil
- 4 cups vegetable broth, low sodium
- 1 tsp balsamic vinegar
- ½ cup basil, fresh, chopped
- 1 tsp oregano, dried
- ½ cup almond milk, unsweetened
- Salt to taste
- Freshly ground black pepper to taste

Directions:

1. Heat olive oil in a pot over medium heat
2. Sauté onion and garlic until translucent, about 5 minutes
3. Add chopped tomatoes and cook for another 10 minutes
4. Pour in vegetable broth, balsamic vinegar, and add oregano
5. Bring to a simmer and cook for 15 minutes
6. Remove from heat, blend until smooth with an immersion blender
7. Return to heat, stir in almond milk and chopped basil, season with salt and pepper, and heat through

Tips:
- Serve with a dollop of Greek yogurt for creaminess without the extra calories
- Garnish with a few basil leaves
- A pinch of chili flakes can add a pleasant heat to the soup

Nutritional Values: Calories: 130, Fat: 5g, Carbs: 18g, Protein: 3g, Sugar: 9g, Sodium: 410 mg, Potassium: 350 mg, Cholesterol: 0 mg

BEEF AND VEGETABLE SOUP

Preparation Time: 20 min - **Cooking Time:** 1 hr 30 min - **Servings:** 6
Glycemic Index: Medium(~64)
Ingredients:
- 1 lb beef stew meat, cubed
- 2 Tbsp olive oil
- 1 onion, chopped
- 3 garlic cloves, minced
- 3 carrots, chopped
- 2 potatoes, peeled and cubed
- ½ cup turnip, peeled and cubed
- 6 cups beef broth, low sodium
- 1 tsp thyme, dried
- Salt to taste

- Freshly ground black pepper to taste
- ½ cup peas, frozen
- 2 Tbsp parsley, fresh, chopped

Directions:

1. Heat olive oil in a large soup pot over medium-high heat
2. Sear beef cubes until browned on all sides, about 5 minutes, then remove and set aside
3. In the same pot, add onion, garlic, carrots, and sauté until onions are translucent
4. Return beef to the pot, add potatoes, turnips, beef broth, thyme, salt, and pepper
5. Bring to a boil, then reduce the heat to low and simmer covered for about 1 hr until meat is tender
6. Stir in peas and cook for an additional 10 minutes
7. Garnish with fresh parsley

Tips:
- Add pearl onions for a burst of sweetness
- Substitute beef broth with low sodium vegetable broth for a lighter variant
- Enhance the flavor with a dash of Worcestershire sauce at the end of cooking

Nutritional Values: Calories: 240, Fat: 9g, Carbs: 20g, Protein: 20g, Sugar: 5g, Sodium: 360 mg, Potassium: 710 mg, Cholesterol: 55 mg

MISO MUSHROOM STEW

Preparation Time: 15 min - **Cooking Time:** 35 min - **Servings:** 4
Glycemic Index: Low(~45)
Ingredients:
- 1 Tbsp olive oil
- 2 cups shiitake mushrooms, sliced
- 1 large onion, chopped
- 2 garlic cloves, minced
- 4 cups vegetable broth, low sodium
- 2 Tbsp miso paste
- 1 Tbsp soy sauce, low sodium
- 1 Tbsp ginger, freshly grated
- 1 cup carrots, julienned
- 1 cup zucchini, julienned
- ½ cup scallions, chopped

Directions:

1. Heat olive oil in a large pot over medium heat
2. Add onions and garlic and sauté until translucent
3. Add mushrooms and cook until they begin to soften

4. In a small bowl, blend miso paste, soy sauce, and a bit of warm broth to create a smooth mixture
5. Add this mixture to the pot along with the remaining broth and ginger
6. Simmer for 25 min
7. Add carrots and zucchini and cook for an additional 10 min
8. Garnish with scallions before serving

Tips:
- Opt for organic miso to maintain a purer flavor
- Enjoy with a side of whole-grain rolls for added fiber

Nutritional Values: Calories: 120, Fat: 4g, Carbs: 18g, Protein: 6g, Sugar: 6g, Sodium: 300 mg, Potassium: 410 mg, Cholesterol: 0 mg

---

7.3. HEALTHY WRAPS AND SANDWICHES

TURKEY AND AVOCADO WRAP

Preparation Time: 15 min - **Cooking Time:** none - **Servings:** 2
Glycemic Index: Low(~45)
Ingredients:
- 2 large whole grain tortillas
- 6 oz. turkey breast, thinly sliced
- 1 ripe avocado, sliced
- 1 C. spinach leaves, fresh
- ½ C. cherry tomatoes, halved
- ¼ C. red onion, thinly sliced
- 2 Tbsp cilantro, fresh, chopped
- 1 Tbsp lime juice
- Salt and pepper to taste

Directions:

1. Lay out the tortillas on a flat surface
2. Spread the avocado slices evenly over each tortilla
3. Drizzle lime juice over the avocados
4. Layer turkey slices, spinach, cherry tomatoes, and red onions on top of the avocado
5. Sprinkle chopped cilantro, salt, and pepper on the fillings
6. Roll each tortilla tightly to encase the fillings, then cut in half diagonally

Tips:
- Opt for low-sodium turkey breast to minimize salt intake
- Press the wrap slightly before cutting to prevent the fillings from falling out

Nutritional Values: Calories: 320, Fat: 13g, Carbs: 28g, Protein: 23g, Sugar: 4g, Sodium: 460 mg, Potassium: 790 mg, Cholesterol: 51 mg

GRILLED VEGGIE SANDWICH

Preparation Time: 20 min - **Cooking Time:** 10 min - **Servings:** 2

Glycemic Index: Low(~52)

Ingredients:

- 4 slices of whole grain bread
- 1 small zucchini, sliced lengthwise
- 1 bell pepper, deseeded and quartered
- 1 small red onion, sliced into rings
- 2 Tbsp olive oil
- 2 Tbsp balsamic vinegar
- ¼ C. goat cheese, crumbled
- Fresh basil leaves
- Salt and pepper to taste

Directions:

1. Brush zucchini, bell pepper, and onion slices with olive oil and balsamic vinegar
2. Season with salt and pepper
3. Grill vegetables on medium heat until tender and charred, about 5 minutes per side
4. Toast the whole grain bread slices lightly
5. Spread goat cheese on one side of each bread slice
6. Layer grilled vegetables and fresh basil on two bread slices, then top with the remaining slices, goat cheese side down

Tips:

- Grill additional vegetables like eggplant or portobello mushrooms for added flavor and texture
- Serve immediately to enjoy the crunchiness of the bread and the creaminess of the goat cheese

Nutritional Values: Calories: 430, Fat: 19g, Carbs: 53g, Protein: 16g, Sugar: 12g, Sodium: 391 mg, Potassium: 644 mg, Cholesterol: 13 mg

CHICKEN CAESAR WRAP

Preparation Time: 20 min - **Cooking Time:** 10 min - **Servings:** 2

Glycemic Index: Low(~48)

Ingredients:

- 2 large whole grain wraps
- 6 oz. chicken breast, grilled and sliced
- 1 C. Romaine lettuce, chopped
- ¼ C. Parmesan cheese, grated
- 2 Tbsp Caesar dressing, low-fat
- 1 tsp Worcestershire sauce
- 1 tsp Dijon mustard
- ½ tsp garlic powder

- Salt and pepper to taste

Directions:

1. Grill chicken breasts seasoned with salt, pepper, and garlic powder until fully cooked, approximately 10 min per side
2. Slice grilled chicken and set aside
3. In a bowl, mix Caesar dressing, Worcestershire sauce, Dijon mustard
4. Lay out the wraps and distribute Romaine lettuce evenly on each
5. Add chicken slices and pour dressing mixture over the chicken
6. Sprinkle Parmesan cheese
7. Roll wraps tightly, and slice diagonally

Tips:

- Use yogurt-based Caesar dressing for a healthier alternative
- Chill the wraps for about 10 min before serving to let flavors meld

Nutritional Values: Calories: 350, Fat: 15g, Carbs: 27g, Protein: 27g, Sugar: 3g, Sodium: 570 mg, Potassium: 450 mg, Cholesterol: 60 mg

TUNA SALAD SANDWICH ON WHOLE GRAIN BREAD

Preparation Time: 15 min - **Cooking Time:** none - **Servings:** 2
Glycemic Index: Low(~47)
Ingredients:

- 4 slices whole grain bread
- 6 oz. canned tuna in water, drained
- 2 Tbsp mayonnaise, low-fat
- 1 celery stalk, finely chopped
- 1 Tbsp red onion, finely chopped
- 1 Tbsp lemon juice
- 1 tsp capers
- ½ tsp dried dill
- Salt and pepper to taste

Directions:

1. In a mixing bowl, combine tuna, mayonnaise, celery, red onion, lemon juice, capers, and dill
2. Season with salt and pepper to taste
3. Mix well to ensure all ingredients are evenly distributed
4. Spread the tuna mixture on two slices of whole grain bread
5. Top with the remaining bread slices

Tips:

- Swap mayonnaise with Greek yogurt for a tangier, healthier twist
- Add a few slices of avocado for extra creaminess and heart-healthy fats

Nutritional Values: Calories: 310, Fat: 9g, Carbs: 32g, Protein: 25g, Sugar: 5g, Sodium: 690 mg, Potassium: 310 mg, Cholesterol: 30 mg

MEDITERRANEAN TUNA AND OLIVE WRAP

Preparation Time: 15 min - **Cooking Time:** none - **Servings:** 2
Glycemic Index: Low(~50)
Ingredients:

- 2 whole grain tortillas
- 1 can (6 oz.) tuna in water, drained
- 1/4 C. kalamata olives, pitted and sliced
- 1/2 red bell pepper, thinly sliced
- 1/4 C. feta cheese, crumbled
- 1/2 C. baby spinach leaves
- 2 Tbsp Greek yogurt
- 1 Tbsp lemon juice
- 1 tsp extra virgin olive oil
- 1/4 tsp black pepper, ground
- 1/4 tsp dried oregano

Directions:

1. Mix tuna, olives, feta cheese, Greek yogurt, lemon juice, olive oil, black pepper, and oregano in a bowl
2. Spread the mixture evenly over the whole grain tortillas
3. Layer thinly sliced red bell pepper and baby spinach leaves on top
4. Roll the tortillas tightly, slice in half, and serve

Tips:

- Opt for yogurt with live cultures for a probiotic boost
- Incorporate a small amount of chopped fresh dill for a herby enhancement
- Ensure tortillas are at room temperature for easier rolling

Nutritional Values: Calories: 310, Fat: 13g, Carbs: 28g, Protein: 22g, Sugar: 4g, Sodium: 580 mg, Potassium: 300 mg, Cholesterol: 35 mg

7.4. LIGHT AND SATISFYING GRAIN BOWLS

BROWN RICE AND VEGGIE BOWL

Preparation Time: 20 min - **Cooking Time:** 25 min - **Servings:** 4
Glycemic Index: Low(~50)
Ingredients:

- 1½ C. brown rice, uncooked
- 3 C. water
- 1 medium bell pepper, diced

- 1 small red onion, finely chopped
- 2 C. broccoli florets
- 1 Tbsp olive oil
- 1 tsp garlic powder
- Salt and pepper to taste
- ¼ C. almonds, sliced
- 1 Tbsp soy sauce, low sodium

Directions:

1. Rinse brown rice under cold water until water runs clear
2. In a medium pot, bring water to a boil and add brown rice, reduce heat to low, cover, and simmer for 25 min until water is absorbed
3. In a large skillet, heat olive oil over medium heat
4. Add red onion and bell pepper, sauté until soft, about 5 min
5. Add broccoli, garlic powder, salt, and pepper, cook until broccoli is vibrant and tender, about 7 min
6. Mix cooked vegetables and rice, add soy sauce, and stir
7. Garnish with sliced almonds

Tips:
- Add a squeeze of fresh lemon juice for a zesty flavor
- Mix in a handful of fresh spinach for added nutrients right before serving

Nutritional Values: Calories: 280, Fat: 9g, Carbs: 44g, Protein: 6g, Sugar: 3g, Sodium: 200 mg, Potassium: 300 mg, Cholesterol: 0 mg

BARLEY AND MUSHROOM BOWL

Preparation Time: 15 min - **Cooking Time:** 40 min - **Servings:** 4
Glycemic Index: Low(~55)
Ingredients:
- 1 C. pearl barley
- 2½ C. vegetable broth
- 1 Tbsp olive oil
- 2 C. mushrooms, sliced
- 1 garlic clove, minced
- 1 tsp thyme, dried
- Salt and pepper to taste
- ½ C. parsley, chopped
- ¼ C. Parmesan cheese, grated

Directions:

1. Rinse barley under cold water until water runs clear

2. In a medium saucepan, bring vegetable broth to a boil, add barley, reduce heat to low, cover, and cook until barley is tender and liquid is absorbed, about 40 min
3. In a skillet, heat olive oil over medium heat
4. Add mushrooms and cook until browned, about 8 min
5. Add garlic and thyme, season with salt and pepper, cook for an additional 2 min
6. Combine cooked barley and mushroom mixture, top with chopped parsley and grated Parmesan cheese

Tips:
- Try roasting the mushrooms in the oven at 375°F (190°C) for a deeper flavor
- Substitute Parmesan with nutritional yeast for a vegan option

Nutritional Values: Calories: 330, Fat: 10g, Carbs: 52g, Protein: 10g, Sugar: 2g, Sodium: 150 mg, Potassium: 280 mg, Cholesterol: 4 mg

FARRO SALAD WITH ROASTED VEGGIES

Preparation Time: 20 min - **Cooking Time:** 30 min - **Servings:** 4
Glycemic Index: Medium(~62)
Ingredients:
- 1 C. farro, rinsed
- 2½ C. water
- 1 small zucchini, cubed
- 1 red bell pepper, cubed
- 1 yellow bell pepper, cubed
- 1 small red onion, sliced
- 2 Tbsp olive oil
- Salt and pepper to taste
- 2 Tbsp balsamic vinegar
- 1 tsp honey
- ½ C. feta cheese, crumbled
- ¼ C. basil leaves, torn

Directions:

1. In a medium pot, cook farro in water until tender and water is absorbed, about 30 min
2. Preheat oven to 425°F (220°C)
3. In a large bowl, toss zucchini, bell peppers, and onion with 1 Tbsp olive oil, salt, and pepper
4. Spread vegetables on a baking sheet and roast until tender and caramelized, about 20 min
5. In a small bowl, whisk together balsamic vinegar, 1 Tbsp olive oil, and honey
6. Combine cooked farro with roasted vegetables, drizzle the dressing and mix well
7. Garnish with feta cheese and basil

Tips:
- Roast additional veggies like carrots or squash for more variety

- Use maple syrup instead of honey for a vegan version

Nutritional Values: Calories: 308, Fat: 12g, Carbs: 45g, Protein: 9g, Sugar: 7g, Sodium: 210 mg, Potassium: 311 mg, Cholesterol: 15 mg

BULGUR AND CHICKPEA BOWL

Preparation Time: 15 min - **Cooking Time:** 20 min - **Servings:** 4

Glycemic Index: Low(~53)

Ingredients:

- 1 C. bulgur
- 2 C. water
- 1 can chickpeas, drained and rinsed
- 1 cucumber, diced
- 1 tomato, diced
- 1 small red onion, finely chopped
- 2 Tbsp olive oil
- Juice of 1 lemon
- 1 tsp cumin
- Salt and pepper to taste
- ¼ C. fresh parsley, chopped

Directions:

1. In a medium pot, bring water to a boil, add bulgur, reduce heat to low, cover, and simmer until tender and water is absorbed, about 15 min
2. In a large bowl, combine cooked bulgur, chickpeas, cucumber, tomato, and red onion
3. In a small bowl, whisk together olive oil, lemon juice, cumin, salt, and pepper to create a dressing
4. Pour dressing over the bulgur mixture, toss to coat evenly
5. Garnish with chopped parsley

Tips:

- Experiment with different herbs like mint or cilantro for a fresh flavor twist
- Add a drizzle of tahini for extra creaminess

Nutritional Values: Calories: 290, Fat: 8g, Carbs: 50g, Protein: 9g, Sugar: 4g, Sodium: 300 mg, Potassium: 410 mg, Cholesterol: 0 mg

QUINOA AND POMEGRANATE DELIGHT BOWL

Preparation Time: 20 min - **Cooking Time:** 15 min - **Servings:** 2

Glycemic Index: Low(~48)

Ingredients:

- 1 C. quinoa, rinsed
- 2 C. water

- 1 pinch sea salt
- 1/2 C. pomegranate seeds
- 1/4 C. fresh mint, chopped
- 1/4 C. feta cheese, crumbled
- 1/4 C. roasted almonds, chopped
- Dressing: 2 Tbsp olive oil
- 1 Tbsp lemon juice
- 1 tsp honey
- 1/2 tsp black pepper, ground

Directions:

1. Place water, quinoa, and sea salt in a medium saucepan and bring to a boil over high heat
2. Reduce heat to low, cover, and simmer for about 15 minutes or until all water is absorbed
3. Remove from heat and let stand for 5 minutes, then fluff with a fork
4. In a small bowl, whisk together olive oil, lemon juice, honey, and black pepper for the dressing
5. Combine cooked quinoa, pomegranate seeds, mint, feta cheese, and roasted almonds in a serving bowl
6. Drizzle the dressing over the bowl and toss gently to combine

Tips:
- Serve immediately while warm, or allow to cool and refrigerate for a refreshing cold salad
- You can substitute cranberries or chopped apple for pomegranate if desired
- Toasting quinoa before boiling enhances its nutty flavor

Nutritional Values: Calories: 335, Fat: 18g, Carbs: 38g, Protein: 8g, Sugar: 7g, Sodium: 115mg, Potassium: 410mg, Cholesterol: 15mg

CHAPTER 8: DINNER RECIPES

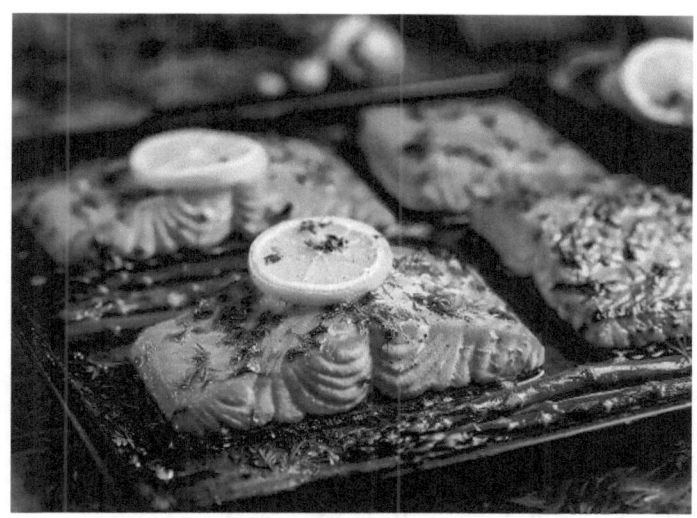

As the sun dips below the horizon and the world settles into the evening, the dinner table becomes a haven, a place where flavors not only meld together but where memories are made. Dinner, in every culture, is more than just a meal; it's a daily coming-together, an opportunity to slow down and share our lives with those we hold dear. For those managing diabetes post-50, this cherished time of day holds even more significance, as it becomes a pivotal moment for nurturing both our bodies and our spirits.

In navigating the landscape of diabetic-friendly cuisine, one might wonder how to retain the soul-satisfying flavors while adhering to a low glycemic diet. That's where the magic of thoughtful preparation and understanding of ingredients comes into play. In this chapter, we make it our mission to convert traditional favorites into dishes that not only respect the dietary needs of those with diabetes but also delight the senses.

Imagine transforming the comforting embrace of a creamy lasagna or the robust zest of a grilled steak into meals that maintain your blood sugar levels without sacrificing taste. Through the recipes provided here, you'll learn how it's entirely possible to indulge in a steaming plate of spicy shrimp curry or savor each bite of a rich, velvety mushroom risotto without the guilt. These recipes are not just about what's left out—no excessive carbs or harmful sugars—but about what's included: wholesomeness, taste, and health.

Moreover, crafting these meals offers a chance to infuse love and care into every dish, an essential ingredient that makes each dinner not merely a routine but a gesture of kindness towards oneself and loved ones. It's about ending your day on a high note, satisfied with the delicious balance on your plate, reassured in the knowledge that your diabetes is well-managed as part of a joyful, vibrant life. As we explore these recipes, let each step and each ingredient be a part of crafting your journey towards health, where every meal is a celebration of life's endless possibilities.

8.1. PROTEIN-RICH MAINS

BAKED SALMON WITH ASPARAGUS

Preparation Time: 15 min - **Cooking Time:** 20 min - **Servings:** 4
Glycemic Index: Low(~40)
Ingredients:

- 4 salmon fillets, 6 oz. each
- 1 lb. asparagus, trimmed
- 2 Tbsp olive oil

- 1 lemon, zest and juice
- 4 cloves garlic, minced
- 1 tsp dried dill
- Salt and pepper to taste

Directions:

1. Preheat oven to 400°F (200°C)
2. Line a baking sheet with foil and place the asparagus on the sheet, drizzle with 1 Tbsp olive oil and sprinkle with salt and pepper
3. Lay the salmon fillets on the asparagus
4. In a small bowl, combine lemon zest and juice, remaining olive oil, garlic, dill, salt, and pepper; whisk well
5. Pour the lemon dill mixture over the salmon
6. Bake in the preheated oven for 20 min or until salmon flakes easily with a fork

Tips:
- Drizzle extra lemon juice for added zestiness
- Serve with a sprinkle of fresh dill or parsley for enhanced aroma

Nutritional Values: Calories: 345, Fat: 23g, Carbs: 6g, Protein: 30g, Sugar: 2g, Sodium: 70 mg, Potassium: 833mg, Cholesterol: 77 mg

CHICKEN STIR-FRY WITH BROCCOLI

Preparation Time: 10 min - **Cooking Time:** 15 min - **Servings:** 4

Glycemic Index: Low(~45)

Ingredients:
- 2 lb. chicken breast, thinly sliced
- 1 lb. broccoli florets
- 1 red bell pepper, julienned
- 2 Tbsp soy sauce, low sodium
- 1 Tbsp sesame oil
- 1 Tbsp ginger, grated
- 2 cloves garlic, minced
- 1 tsp cornstarch
- ¼ cup chicken broth, low sodium

Directions:

1. Heat sesame oil in a large skillet over medium-high heat
2. Add chicken and cook until browned, about 5-7 min, remove from skillet
3. In the same skillet, add broccoli and bell pepper, stir-fry for about 3 min
4. Add ginger and garlic, stir-fry for another 2 min
5. In a small bowl, mix chicken broth, soy sauce, and cornstarch, pour over the vegetables, bring to a simmer

6. Return chicken to skillet, combine and cook until the sauce thickens and chicken is cooked through, about 5 min

Tips:

- Consider adding a splash of hoisin sauce for a slight sweetness
- Garnish with sesame seeds or sliced green onions for a refreshing crunch

Nutritional Values: Calories: 280, Fat: 8g, Carbs: 10g, Protein: 40g, Sugar: 3g, Sodium: 220 mg, Potassium: 890 mg, Cholesterol: 98 mg

GRILLED TOFU WITH VEGETABLES

Preparation Time: 25 min - **Cooking Time:** 15 min - **Servings:** 4
Glycemic Index: Low(~40)
Ingredients:

- 16 oz. firm tofu, pressed and sliced into 1-inch cubes
- 1 zucchini, sliced
- 1 yellow squash, sliced
- 1 red onion, cut into wedges
- 1 red bell pepper, sliced
- 2 Tbsp olive oil
- 1 tsp smoked paprika
- 1 tsp garlic powder
- Salt and pepper to taste

Directions:

1. Preheat grill to medium-high heat (around 375°F or 190°C)
2. In a large bowl, toss tofu and vegetables with olive oil, smoked paprika, garlic powder, salt, and pepper
3. Thread tofu and vegetables alternately onto skewers
4. Grill on preheated grill, turning occasionally, until vegetables are tender and tofu is slightly charred, about 15 min

Tips:

- Brush with a balsamic glaze before serving for an extra layer of flavor
- Pair with a quinoa salad for a complete meal
- If wooden skewers are used, soak them in water for 30 min prior to grilling to prevent burning

Nutritional Values: Calories: 200, Fat: 12g, Carbs: 15g, Protein: 12g, Sugar: 6g, Sodium: 54 mg, Potassium: 512 mg, Cholesterol: 0 mg

BEEF TENDERLOIN WITH GARLIC GREEN BEANS

Preparation Time: 20 min - **Cooking Time:** 30 min - **Servings:** 4
Glycemic Index: Low(~45)

Ingredients:
- 2 lb. beef tenderloin
- 1 lb. green beans, trimmed
- 4 cloves garlic, minced
- 2 Tbsp olive oil
- 1 Tbsp rosemary, chopped
- Salt and pepper to taste

Directions:
1. Preheat oven to 375°F (190°C)
2. Rub the beef tenderloin with 1 Tbsp olive oil, chopped rosemary, salt, and pepper
3. Place in a roasting pan and roast for about 25-30 min for medium-rare (internal temperature should reach 145°F or 63°C)
4. Meanwhile, heat the remaining olive oil in a skillet, add green beans and garlic, sauté until the beans are bright green and slightly tender, about 7 min

Tips:
- Let the beef rest for 10 min before slicing to retain juices
- Serve green beans alongside the sliced tenderloin, drizzle with the pan juices for added flavor

Nutritional Values: Calories: 395, Fat: 20g, Carbs: 10g, Protein: 45g, Sugar: 3g, Sodium: 67 mg, Potassium: 904 mg, Cholesterol: 135 mg

ZESTY LIME SHRIMP AND AVOCADO SALAD

Preparation Time: 15 min - **Cooking Time:** 10 min - **Servings:** 4
Glycemic Index: Low(~30)
Ingredients:
- 1 lb shrimp, peeled and deveined
- 2 avocados, diced
- 1 medium red onion, finely chopped
- 2 tomatoes, diced
- 1 jalapeno, seeded and finely chopped
- 1/4 C. cilantro, chopped
- Juice of 2 limes
- 1 Tbsp olive oil
- Salt and black pepper to taste

Directions:
1. Season shrimp with salt and black pepper
2. Heat olive oil in a skillet over medium heat and sauté shrimp until pink and cooked through, about 5-7 minutes
3. In a large bowl, combine cooked shrimp, avocados, red onion, tomatoes, jalapeno, and cilantro
4. Drizzle with lime juice and toss gently to mix

Tips:
- Serve immediately and enjoy cold for a refreshing taste
- Add a pinch of cumin for an extra kick of flavor

Nutritional Values: Calories: 250, Fat: 15g, Carbs: 12g, Protein: 20g, Sugar: 2g, Sodium: 210 mg, Potassium: 450 mg, Cholesterol: 180 mg

---

8.2. Vegetable-Centric Dishes

Stuffed Bell Peppers with Quinoa

Preparation Time: 15 min - **Cooking Time:** 40 min - **Servings:** 4

Glycemic Index: Low(~50)

Ingredients:
- 4 large bell peppers, tops cut off and seeds removed
- 1 cup quinoa, rinsed
- 2 cups vegetable broth
- 1 tbsp olive oil
- 1 onion, finely chopped
- 2 garlic cloves, minced
- 1 zucchini, diced
- 1 carrot, grated
- 1 tsp dried oregano
- 1 tsp dried basil
- 1/2 tsp salt
- 1/4 tsp black pepper
- 1/2 cup tomatoes, diced
- 1/2 cup low-fat feta cheese, crumbled

Directions:

1. Preheat oven to 375°F (190°C)
2. In a saucepan, bring the vegetable broth to a boil and add quinoa, reduce heat and simmer covered until liquid is absorbed and quinoa is tender, about 15 min
3. In a skillet, heat olive oil and sauté onion and garlic until translucent, add zucchini and carrot, cooking until soft
4. Combine cooked quinoa with sautéed vegetables, oregano, basil, salt, pepper, and tomatoes
5. Spoon the mixture into hollowed-out bell peppers, top each with feta cheese
6. Place stuffed peppers upright in a baking dish, cover with foil, and bake for 25 min, uncover and bake for an additional 15 min until peppers are tender and cheese is golden brown

Tips:
- Consider using different colors of bell peppers for visual appeal
- Substitute quinoa with bulgur for a variation in texture

- Add pine nuts for a crunchy texture

Nutritional Values: Calories: 292, Fat: 9g, Carbs: 44g, Protein: 12g, Sugar: 9g, Sodium: 307 mg, Potassium: 670 mg, Cholesterol: 8 mg

EGGPLANT PARMESAN (LOW GLYCEMIC)

Preparation Time: 20 min - **Cooking Time:** 45 min - **Servings:** 4

Glycemic Index: Low(~45)

Ingredients:

- 2 large eggplants, sliced into 1/2-inch thick rounds
- 1 tsp salt
- 2 cups marinara sauce, low sodium
- 1 cup shredded mozzarella, low-fat
- 1/2 cup Parmesan cheese, grated
- 1/4 cup fresh basil, chopped
- 1 tbsp olive oil
- 3 garlic cloves, minced
- 1/2 tsp black pepper

Directions:

1. Salt eggplant slices and let sit for 10 min to draw out bitterness, rinse and pat dry
2. Preheat oven to 400°F (204°C)
3. In a skillet, heat olive oil and sauté garlic until fragrant
4. Layer the bottom of a baking dish with half of the marinara sauce, place a layer of eggplant slices, top with half of the mozzarella and Parmesan, and sprinkle with basil, repeat layers
5. Cover with foil and bake for 30 min, remove foil and bake for another 15 min until cheese is bubbly and golden

Tips:

- Use a paper towel to remove excess moisture from the eggplant after rinsing for crisper layers
- For added flavor, incorporate a layer of thinly sliced zucchini

Nutritional Values: Calories: 274, Fat: 16g, Carbs: 22g, Protein: 17g, Sugar: 11g, Sodium: 474 mg, Potassium: 717 mg, Cholesterol: 22 mg

ROASTED CAULIFLOWER STEAKS

Preparation Time: 10 min - **Cooking Time:** 25 min - **Servings:** 4

Glycemic Index: Low(~30)

Ingredients:

- 1 large head cauliflower, sliced into 1-inch thick steaks
- 2 tbsp olive oil
- 1 tsp smoked paprika
- 1/2 tsp garlic powder

- 1/2 tsp onion powder
- 1/4 tsp salt
- 1/4 tsp black pepper
- 1 lemon, juiced
- 2 tbsp parsley, chopped

Directions:

1. Preheat oven to 425°F (218°C)
2. Brush both sides of each cauliflower steak with olive oil and season with smoked paprika, garlic powder, onion powder, salt, and pepper
3. Arrange cauliflower steaks on a baking sheet in a single layer
4. Roast in the preheated oven for 12 min, flip steaks, and continue roasting until golden and tender, about 13 min more
5. Drizzle with lemon juice and garnish with parsley before serving

Tips:
- For a charred flavor, broil cauliflower steaks for the last 2 min of roasting
- Serve with a tahini drizzle for an extra layer of flavor

Nutritional Values: Calories: 123, Fat: 7g, Carbs: 13g, Protein: 5g, Sugar: 5g, Sodium: 319 mg, Potassium: 640 mg, Cholesterol: 0 mg

ZUCCHINI NOODLES WITH PESTO

Preparation Time: 10 min - **Cooking Time:** 5 min - **Servings:** 4
Glycemic Index: Low(~45)
Ingredients:
- 4 medium zucchinis, spiralized
- 1 cup fresh basil leaves
- 1/4 cup pine nuts
- 2 garlic cloves
- 1/4 cup Parmesan cheese, grated
- 1/4 cup olive oil
- Salt and pepper to taste

Directions:

1. In a food processor, combine basil, pine nuts, garlic, and Parmesan cheese, pulse until coarse meal forms
2. With processor running, slowly add olive oil until smooth pesto forms, season with salt and pepper
3. In a skillet, sauté spiralized zucchini noodles for about 3-5 min until tender
4. Remove from heat and toss with prepared pesto

Tips:
- Serve immediately for best texture
- Top with additional Parmesan cheese if desired
- For a protein boost, add grilled chicken or shrimp

Nutritional Values: Calories: 262, Fat: 22g, Carbs: 14g, Protein: 6g, Sugar: 4g, Sodium: 210 mg, Potassium: 512 mg, Cholesterol: 4 mg

MEDITERRANEAN STUFFED ARTICHOKES

Preparation Time: 20 min - **Cooking Time:** 45 min - **Servings:** 4

Glycemic Index: Low(~45)

Ingredients:
- 4 large artichokes, halved and chokes removed
- 1 C. quinoa, cooked
- 1/2 C. feta cheese, crumbled
- 1/4 C. olives, chopped
- 1/4 C. sun-dried tomatoes, chopped
- 2 Tbsp pine nuts, toasted
- 2 cloves garlic, minced
- 2 Tbsp olive oil
- 1 tsp lemon zest
- Juice of one lemon
- 1/2 tsp each of dried basil, oregano, and black pepper

Directions:

1. Preheat oven to 375°F (190°C)
2. In a bowl, combine quinoa, feta, olives, sun-dried tomatoes, pine nuts, and garlic
3. Mix in olive oil, lemon zest, lemon juice, and herbs; stir to combine
4. Fill each artichoke half with the quinoa mixture
5. Place stuffed artichokes in a baking dish and cover with foil
6. Bake covered for 30 min, then uncover and bake for an additional 15 min or until tops are slightly golden and artichokes are tender

Tips:
- Drizzle with extra virgin olive oil before serving for added richness
- Squeeze additional lemon juice on top for a zesty flavor
- Can be served either warm or at room temperature for convenience

Nutritional Values: Calories: 250, Fat: 15g, Carbs: 23g, Protein: 8g, Sugar: 3g, Sodium: 420 mg, Potassium: 350 mg, Cholesterol: 25 mg

QUINOA AND CHICKEN CASSEROLE

Preparation Time: 20 min - **Cooking Time:** 45 min - **Servings:** 4

Glycemic Index: Low(~40)

Ingredients:

- 1 C. quinoa, rinsed
- 2 C. low-sodium chicken broth
- 1 lb chicken breast, cubed
- 1 C. carrots, diced
- 1 C. bell peppers, chopped
- 2 cloves garlic, minced
- 1 tsp turmeric powder
- 1 tsp smoked paprika
- ½ tsp black pepper
- 1 C. spinach, fresh
- ½ C. low-fat feta cheese, crumbled

Directions:

1. Preheat oven to 375°F (190°C)
2. In a large bowl, mix quinoa, chicken broth, turmeric, paprika, and black pepper
3. Spread the quinoa mixture at the bottom of a baking dish
4. Layer chicken, carrots, bell peppers, and garlic on top
5. Cover with foil and bake for 40 min
6. Uncover, add spinach and feta, bake for an additional 5 min

Tips:

- Add a squeeze of lemon for a tangy twist
- Top with fresh parsley for added freshness
- Serve with a side of steamed green beans for a complete meal

Nutritional Values: Calories: 450, Fat: 12g, Carbs: 48g, Protein: 36g, Sugar: 5g, Sodium: 300 mg, Potassium: 800 mg, Cholesterol: 75 mg

VEGETABLE AND LENTIL CURRY

Preparation Time: 15 min - **Cooking Time:** 30 min - **Servings:** 4

Glycemic Index: Low(~45)

Ingredients:

- 1 C. red lentils, rinsed
- 1 onion, diced
- 2 C. low-sodium vegetable broth
- 1 C. cauliflower florets

- 1 C. green beans, trimmed and halved
- 2 Tbsp curry powder
- 1 tsp cumin powder
- 1 can (14.5 oz) diced tomatoes, no salt added
- 1 C. coconut milk
- 1 Tbsp ginger, grated
- 1 tsp olive oil

Directions:

1. Heat olive oil in a large pot over medium heat
2. Sauté onion with ginger until translucent
3. Stir in curry and cumin powder, cooking for 1 min
4. Add lentils, vegetable broth, cauliflower, green beans, and tomatoes
5. Bring to a boil, reduce heat and simmer covered for 25 min
6. Stir in coconut milk and heat through for another 5 min

Tips:
- Serve over a small portion of brown rice for extra fiber
- Garnish with fresh cilantro for a burst of flavor
- Add a splash of lime juice for extra zing

Nutritional Values: Calories: 295, Fat: 9g, Carbs: 38g, Protein: 15g, Sugar: 6g, Sodium: 250 mg, Potassium: 850 mg, Cholesterol: 0 mg

TURKEY AND SWEET POTATO SKILLET

Preparation Time: 10 min - **Cooking Time:** 20 min - **Servings:** 4
Glycemic Index: Low(~50)
Ingredients:
- 1 lb turkey breast, ground
- 2 C. sweet potatoes, cubed
- 1 onion, chopped
- 1 red bell pepper, diced
- 2 cloves garlic, minced
- 1 tsp chili powder
- 1 tsp cumin
- ½ tsp salt
- ½ tsp black pepper
- 2 Tbsp olive oil
- 1 C. kale, chopped
- ¼ C. water

Directions:

1. Heat olive oil in a large skillet over medium-high heat

2. Add turkey and sauté until browned
3. Add onion, bell pepper, garlic, chili powder, cumin, salt, and pepper, cooking until vegetables are soft
4. Add sweet potatoes and water, cover, reduce heat to medium-low and simmer until potatoes are tender, about 15 min
5. Stir in kale and cook until wilted

Tips:
- Opt for lean turkey to reduce fat content
- Serve with whole-wheat tortillas for a hearty wrap
- Sprinkle with freshly grated low-fat cheese for extra flavor

Nutritional Values: Calories: 320, Fat: 10g, Carbs: 30g, Protein: 25g, Sugar: 7g, Sodium: 350 mg, Potassium: 900 mg, Cholesterol: 55 mg

SHRIMP AND BROWN RICE PAELLA

Preparation Time: 15 min - **Cooking Time:** 35 min - **Servings:** 4
Glycemic Index: Low(~55)

Ingredients:
- 1 C. brown rice, uncooked
- 1 lb shrimp, peeled and deveined
- 1 onion, diced
- 2 tomatoes, diced
- 1 bell pepper, chopped
- 2 cloves garlic, minced
- 1 tsp saffron threads
- 1 tsp smoked paprika
- ½ tsp salt
- ½ C. frozen peas
- 3 C. low-sodium fish broth
- 2 Tbsp olive oil

Directions:

1. Heat olive oil in a large skillet or paella pan over medium heat
2. Sauté onion and garlic until translucent
3. Add tomatoes, bell pepper, and paprika, cook for 5 min
4. Stir in rice, saffron, salt, and broth
5. Bring to a boil, then reduce to a simmer, cover and cook until rice is tender, about 25 min
6. Stir in shrimp and peas, cook until shrimp are pink and cooked through, about 10 more min

Tips:
- Serve with a wedge of lemon for extra zest
- Garnish with chopped parsley for color and freshness

- For a low sodium version, substitute water for some of the broth

Nutritional Values: Calories: 410, Fat: 12g, Carbs: 52g, Protein: 28g, Sugar: 4g, Sodium: 300 mg, Potassium: 600 mg, Cholesterol: 180 mg

MEDITERRANEAN CHICKEN AND QUINOA STEW

Preparation Time: 15 min - **Cooking Time:** 30 min - **Servings:** 4

Glycemic Index: Low(~50)

Ingredients:

- 2 Tbsp olive oil
- 1 lb chicken breast, cubed
- 1 onion, finely chopped
- 3 cloves garlic, minced
- 1 red bell pepper, diced
- 1 zucchini, diced
- 1 C. quinoa, rinsed
- 2 C. chicken broth, low sodium
- 1 can (14 oz.) diced tomatoes, no salt added
- 1 tsp dried oregano
- 1 tsp dried basil
- Salt and pepper to taste

Directions:

1. Heat olive oil in a large pot over medium heat
2. Add chicken and brown on all sides, then set aside
3. In the same pot, sauté onion and garlic until translucent
4. Add bell pepper and zucchini and cook for another 5 min
5. Return chicken to the pot along with quinoa, broth, diced tomatoes, oregano, and basil
6. Bring to a boil, then cover and simmer for 20 min or until quinoa is cooked
7. Season with salt and pepper before serving

Tips:

- Serve with a sprinkle of fresh parsley for a fresh touch
- Accompany with a side of mixed greens for a complete meal

Nutritional Values: Calories: 410, Fat: 12g, Carbs: 43g, Protein: 33g, Sugar: 7g, Sodium: 300 mg, Potassium: 960 mg, Cholesterol: 65 mg

8.4. WHOLE GRAIN PASTA AND RICE DISHES

WHOLE WHEAT SPAGHETTI WITH MARINARA

Preparation Time: 15 min - **Cooking Time:** 20 min - **Servings:** 4
Glycemic Index: Low(~45)
Ingredients:

- 12 oz. whole wheat spaghetti
- 2 cups marinara sauce, low-sodium
- 1 Tbsp olive oil
- 1 clove garlic, minced
- 1 tsp dried basil
- 1 tsp dried oregano
- 1 pinch salt, optional
- 1 pinch black pepper

Directions:

1. Bring a large pot of water to a boil, add a pinch of salt, and cook spaghetti according to package instructions
2. In a separate saucepan, heat olive oil over medium heat, sauté garlic until fragrant, about 1 min
3. Add marinara sauce, basil, and oregano, simmer for 15 min, stirring occasionally
4. Drain spaghetti and combine with the sauce, season with salt and pepper to taste

Tips:

- Use fresh basil leaves as garnish for enhanced aroma and a touch of freshness
- Stir in some red pepper flakes if you like a bit of spice in your meals

Nutritional Values: Calories: 320, Fat: 4.5g, Carbs: 61g, Protein: 10g, Sugar: 4g, Sodium: 210 mg, Potassium: 380 mg, Cholesterol: 0 mg

BROWN RICE PILAF WITH HERBS

Preparation Time: 10 min - **Cooking Time:** 35 min - **Servings:** 4
Glycemic Index: Low(~55)
Ingredients:

- 2 cups brown rice
- 4 cups water
- 1 Tbsp olive oil
- 1 medium onion, finely chopped
- 1 clove garlic, minced
- 1 tsp thyme, dried
- 1 tsp rosemary, dried
- 1/4 cup parsley, freshly chopped

- Salt and pepper, to taste

Directions:

1. In a saucepan, heat olive oil over medium heat, add onion and garlic and sauté until onion is translucent
2. Add brown rice to the pan and stir for 2 min to lightly toast the grains
3. Add water, thyme, and rosemary, bring to a boil, then reduce to a simmer, cover, and cook until water is absorbed and rice is tender, about 30 min
4. Remove from heat, stir in parsley, and season with salt and pepper

Tips:

- Before serving, fluff with a fork to separate the grains for a better texture
- Lemon zest can be added for a refreshing twist

Nutritional Values: Calories: 216, Fat: 3.5g, Carbs: 40g, Protein: 5g, Sugar: 1g, Sodium: 10 mg, Potassium: 150 mg, Cholesterol: 0 mg

QUINOA PRIMAVERA

Preparation Time: 15 min - **Cooking Time:** 20 min - **Servings:** 4

Glycemic Index: Low(~50)

Ingredients:

- 2 cups quinoa, rinsed
- 4 cups vegetable broth, low-sodium
- 1 Tbsp olive oil
- 1/2 bell pepper, chopped
- 1 zucchini, diced
- 1/2 cup cherry tomatoes, halved
- 1/4 cup carrots, diced
- 1/2 tsp garlic powder
- 1/2 tsp onion powder
- 1 Tbsp parsley, chopped
- Salt and pepper, to taste

Directions:

1. In a large pot, bring quinoa and vegetable broth to a boil, then reduce to a simmer, cover and cook until quinoa is fluffy and transparent, about 15 min
2. Meanwhile, heat olive oil in a skillet, add bell pepper, zucchini, cherry tomatoes, and carrots, sauté until vegetables are tender, about 7 min
3. Combine cooked quinoa with the sautéed vegetables, add garlic powder, onion powder, parsley, and season with salt and pepper

Tips:

- Serve warm with a slice of lemon for added zest

- Sprinkle nutritional yeast for a cheesy flavor without the dairy

Nutritional Values: Calories: 295, Fat: 5g, Carbs: 53g, Protein: 11g, Sugar: 3g, Sodium: 300 mg, Potassium: 430 mg, Cholesterol: 0 mg

BARLEY RISOTTO WITH MUSHROOMS

Preparation Time: 15 min - **Cooking Time:** 40 min - **Servings:** 4

Glycemic Index: Low(~53)

Ingredients:
- 1 cup pearl barley, rinsed
- 4 cups vegetable stock, low-sodium
- 1 Tbsp olive oil
- 1 cup mushrooms, sliced
- 1 small onion, diced
- 1 clove garlic, minced
- 1/4 cup Parmesan cheese, grated
- 1 tsp thyme, dried
- Salt and pepper, to taste

Directions:

1. Heat olive oil in a large pan, sauté onions and garlic for about 3 min until onion turns translucent
2. Add mushrooms and cook until they're browned and have released their juices, about 10 min
3. Stir in barley and add one cup of vegetable stock, stir continuously until absorbed, continue adding stock one cup at a time until barley is creamy and al dente about 25 min
4. Mix in Parmesan cheese, thyme, salt, and pepper

Tips:
- Sprinkle with chopped parsley for a pop of color and freshness
- For a vegan option, substitute Parmesan with nutritional yeast

Nutritional Values: Calories: 345, Fat: 7g, Carbs: 59g, Protein: 12g, Sugar: 2g, Sodium: 240 mg, Potassium: 280 mg, Cholesterol: 4 mg

MEDITERRANEAN FARRO SALAD WITH GRILLED VEGETABLES

Preparation Time: 15 min - **Cooking Time:** 25 min - **Servings:** 4

Glycemic Index: Low(~45)

Ingredients:
- 1 C. farro
- 1 medium zucchini, sliced vertically
- 1 red bell pepper, cut into quarters
- 1 small red onion, sliced into rings
- 2 Tbsp olive oil

- 2 cloves garlic, minced
- ⅓ C. feta cheese, crumbled
- ¼ C. fresh basil leaves, chopped
- 2 Tbsp balsamic vinegar
- Salt and pepper to taste

Directions:

1. Rinse farro under cold water and cook as per package instructions until al dente
2. Preheat grill to medium-high (375°F / 190°C)
3. Toss zucchini, bell pepper, and onion with olive oil, and garlic in a bowl, season with salt and pepper
4. Grill vegetables for about 12 min, turning occasionally until tender and charred
5. Chop grilled vegetables and toss with cooked farro, feta cheese, basil, and balsamic vinegar

Tips:

- Add a sprinkle of dried oregano for a more robust flavor
- Grill vegetables in a grill basket to prevent slices from falling through the grates

Nutritional Values: Calories: 353, Fat: 14g, Carbs: 48g, Protein: 10g, Sugar: 6g, Sodium: 276 mg, Potassium: 342 mg, Cholesterol: 16 mg

CHAPTER 9: SMART SNACKING

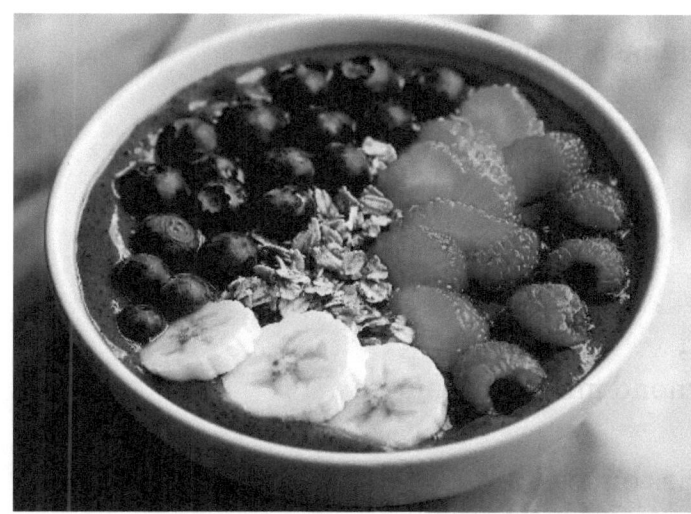

Ah, the art of snacking—often seen as the pitfall of many well-intentioned diets, yet it offers an unheralded pathway to sustaining balanced blood sugar levels and replenishing energy, especially in the life of someone managing diabetes post-50. Now, when it comes to diabetes, the mantra often sung is about strict meal schedules and rigorous adherence to balanced meals. However, what if I told you that smart snacking isn't just permissible but can indeed be a cornerstone of maintaining a healthy and enjoyable diet plan?

Imagine this: It's midafternoon; lunch feels like a distant memory, and dinner is still a horizon away. Your stomach rumbles, and you're faced with a decision that could either support your health goals or set you back. Here is where the unsung heroes of the diabetic world come into play—the smart snacks.

Smart snacking is far from digging into the nearest bag of chips. It involves strategic choices that stabilize your blood sugar and keep those pesky hunger pangs at bay without compromising your flavor palette. It's about turning to snacks that are rich in fiber, good fats, and protein—all of which are comrades in your quest to manage diabetes effectively.

But, let's make this practical. Picture yourself reaching for a small bowl of greek yogurt topped with a handful of antioxidant-rich berries and a sprinkle of chia seeds – a delightful, creamy medley that not only satisfies those urgent hunger knocks but also keeps the blood sugar checks in balance. Or consider a crisp apple with a smear of almond butter, a snack that pairs the natural sweetness of fruit with the creamy, protein-packed goodness of nuts.

This chapter isn't just a collection of recipes; it's a new narrative in your diabetic management story where snacking is not a guilty pleasure but a healthful necessity. Perfectly crafted to nurture your body between meals, these snacking ideas are poised to add not just nutritional value but also moments of simple pleasures to your everyday routine—a testament to the fact that living well with diabetes can indeed be delicious and satisfying. So, let us embark on this tasty snacking journey together, ensuring each bite is not only delightful but also aligned perfectly with your health goals.

9.1. NUTRITIOUS SMOOTHIE BOWLS

ACAI BOWL WITH BERRIES

Preparation Time: 10 min - **Cooking Time:** none - **Servings:** 2
Glycemic Index: Low(~46)

Ingredients:

- 1 pack acai berry puree, unsweetened
- 1 C. mixed berries (blueberries, strawberries, and raspberries)
- 1 banana, sliced
- ½ C. granola, low-sugar
- 1 Tbsp almond butter
- ¼ C. almond milk, unsweetened

Directions:

1. Thaw the acai puree slightly for easy blending
2. Blend acai puree with half the banana and almond milk until smooth
3. Pour mixture into bowls
4. Arrange remaining banana slices, mixed berries on top
5. Drizzle with almond butter and sprinkle granola over everything

Tips:

- To boost protein, add a scoop of vanilla whey protein isolate to the blend
- Opt for homemade granola to control sugar content
- Garnish with a few mint leaves for a refreshing touch

Nutritional Values: Calories: 325, Fat: 12g, Carbs: 47g, Protein: 6g, Sugar: 28g, Sodium: 65 mg, Potassium: 366 mg, Cholesterol: 0 mg

GREEN SMOOTHIE BOWL WITH KIWI

Preparation Time: 15 min - **Cooking Time:** none - **Servings:** 1
Glycemic Index: Low(~49)

Ingredients:

- 2 ripe kiwis, peeled and sliced
- 1 C. baby spinach
- ½ avocado
- ½ C. Greek yogurt, low-fat
- 1 Tbsp honey, optional
- 2 Tbsp chia seeds
- ½ C. coconut water

Directions:

1. Blend spinach, one kiwi, avocado, Greek yogurt, and coconut water until smooth
2. Pour into a bowl
3. Top with sliced kiwi, chia seeds, and a drizzle of honey if using

Tips:

- Add a pinch of spirulina or matcha powder for a superfood boost
- Use agave syrup instead of honey for a lower GI sweetener

- Serve immediately to maintain optimum freshness and texture

Nutritional Values: Calories: 295, Fat: 15g, Carbs: 35g, Protein: 8g, Sugar: 20g, Sodium: 42 mg, Potassium: 782 mg, Cholesterol: 2.5 mg

TROPICAL SMOOTHIE BOWL WITH COCONUT

Preparation Time: 12 min - **Cooking Time:** none - **Servings:** 2

Glycemic Index: Medium(~56)

Ingredients:

- ½ C. mango, chopped
- ½ C. pineapple, chopped
- 1 banana, sliced
- 1/3 C. coconut milk, lite
- Tbsp coconut flakes, unsweetened
- ¼ C. vanilla Greek yogurt, low-fat
- 1 Tbsp flaxseed, ground

Directions:

1. Blend mango, pineapple, half the banana, coconut milk, and Greek yogurt until creamy
2. Pour mixture into bowls
3. Top with remaining banana slices, and sprinkle with coconut flakes and ground flaxseed

Tips:

- Freeze the fruits in advance for a thicker, ice-cream like consistency
- Choose unsweetened coconut flakes to minimize added sugars
- Drizzle with a little lime juice for a tangy flavor enhancement

Nutritional Values: Calories: 330, Fat: 9g, Carbs: 56g, Protein: 6g, Sugar: 38g, Sodium: 30 mg, Potassium: 524 mg, Cholesterol: 1 mg

PROTEIN-RICH BERRY BOWL

Preparation Time: 15 min - **Cooking Time:** none - **Servings:** 2

Glycemic Index: Low(~45)

Ingredients:

- ½ C. raspberries
- ½ C. blackberries
- 1 C. cottage cheese, low-fat
- 1 Tbsp pumpkin seeds
- 2 Tbsp honey, optional
- 1 Tbsp hemp seeds
- ½ C. almond milk, unsweetened

Directions:

1. Blend cottage cheese, almond milk, and half the berries until smooth

2. Spread this creamy base in two bowls
3. Top with remaining berries, pumpkin seeds, and hemp seeds
4. Drizzle honey over each bowl if desired

Tips:
- Mix in a scoop of low-GI protein powder for added protein
- Swap honey with a diabetic-friendly sweetener if sugar is a concern
- Stir in a spoonful of almond butter for extra richness and satiety

Nutritional Values: Calories: 280, Fat: 10g, Carbs: 32g, Protein: 19g, Sugar: 22g, Sodium: 105 mg, Potassium: 217 mg, Cholesterol: 5 mg

SPICED PUMPKIN SMOOTHIE BOWL

Preparation Time: 10 min - **Cooking Time:** none - **Servings:** 1
Glycemic Index: Low(~35)
Ingredients:
- 1 C. pumpkin purée
- 1/2 C. Greek yogurt, low-fat
- 1/4 C. rolled oats
- 1 Tbsp almond butter
- 1/2 tsp cinnamon
- 1/4 tsp nutmeg
- 1/2 tsp vanilla extract
- 1/4 C. almond milk, unsweetened
- 1 tsp pumpkin seeds for garnish
- 1/2 apple, finely diced

Directions:
1. Blend pumpkin purée, Greek yogurt, rolled oats, almond butter, cinnamon, nutmeg, vanilla extract, and almond milk until smooth
2. Pour into a bowl and garnish with pumpkin seeds and diced apple

Tips:
- Add a dash of ground ginger for a warm spice note
- Opt for freshly ground nutmeg for more potent flavor

Nutritional Values: Calories: 315, Fat: 10g, Carbs: 45g, Protein: 12g, Sugar: 18g, Sodium: 60 mg, Potassium: 300 mg, Cholesterol: 5 mg

ROASTED CHICKPEAS

Preparation Time: 10 min - **Cooking Time:** 30 min - **Servings:** 4

Glycemic Index: Low(~55)

Ingredients:

- 1 can chickpeas, rinsed and dried
- 1 Tbsp olive oil
- 1 tsp smoked paprika
- 1/2 tsp garlic powder
- 1/4 tsp cayenne pepper
- Salt to taste
- 1/2 tsp cumin

Directions:

1. Preheat oven to 400°F (204°C)
2. Toss chickpeas with olive oil, smoked paprika, garlic powder, cayenne pepper, salt, and cumin in a bowl until evenly coated
3. Spread chickpeas on a baking sheet in a single layer
4. Roast in the oven for 30 min, shaking the pan every 10 min to ensure even cooking

Tips:

- Store in an airtight container to maintain crunchiness
- Adjust spices based on personal preference for heat and flavor

Nutritional Values: Calories: 210, Fat: 6g, Carbs: 30g, Protein: 10g, Sugar: 5g, Sodium: 300 mg, Potassium: 290 mg, Cholesterol: 0 mg

SPICED NUTS MIX

Preparation Time: 15 min - **Cooking Time:** 20 min - **Servings:** 6

Glycemic Index: Low(~40)

Ingredients:

- 1 cup almonds
- 1 cup walnuts
- 1 cup pecans
- 1 Tbsp olive oil
- 1 tsp chili powder
- 1/2 tsp cinnamon
- 1/4 tsp nutmeg
- 1 tsp sea salt
- 1/2 tsp black pepper

Directions:

1. Preheat oven to 350°F (177°C)
2. Mix almonds, walnuts, and pecans with olive oil in a large bowl
3. Add chili powder, cinnamon, nutmeg, sea salt, and black pepper and toss to coat evenly
4. Spread nuts on a baking sheet and bake for 20 min, stirring occasionally

Tips:

- Can be served warm or at room temperature for enhanced flavor profiles
- Experiment with different spices like curry powder or cumin for variety
- Store in a cool, dry place in an airtight container

Nutritional Values: Calories: 320, Fat: 28g, Carbs: 12g, Protein: 8g, Sugar: 2g, Sodium: 340 mg, Potassium: 380 mg, Cholesterol: 0 mg

BAKED ZUCCHINI CHIPS

Preparation Time: 15 min - **Cooking Time:** 2 hr - **Servings:** 3
Glycemic Index: Low(~42)
Ingredients:

- 2 large zucchinis, thinly sliced
- 1 Tbsp olive oil
- 1 tsp sea salt
- 1/2 tsp black pepper
- 1 tsp dried oregano
- 1 tsp dried basil

Directions:

1. Preheat oven to 225°F (107°C)
2. Toss thinly sliced zucchinis with olive oil, sea salt, black pepper, oregano, and basil
3. Arrange slices in a single layer on a baking sheet lined with parchment paper
4. Bake for 2 hr, turning slices halfway through until crisp

Tips:

- Use a mandolin slicer for evenly thin slices
- Pat zucchini slices dry with a paper towel before seasoning to ensure crispiness

Nutritional Values: Calories: 50, Fat: 3.5g, Carbs: 4g, Protein: 1.5g, Sugar: 3g, Sodium: 580 mg, Potassium: 310 mg, Cholesterol: 0 mg

KALE CHIPS WITH SEA SALT

Preparation Time: 10 min - **Cooking Time:** 15 min - **Servings:** 4
Glycemic Index: Low(~40)
Ingredients:

- 1 bunch kale, stems removed and leaves torn
- 1 Tbsp olive oil

- 1 tsp sea salt

Directions:

1. Preheat oven to 350°F (177°C)
2. Toss kale leaves with olive oil and sea salt in a bowl until evenly coated
3. Spread kale leaves on a baking sheet in a single layer
4. Bake for 15 min or until edges are brown but not burnt

Tips:
- Massage kale leaves with olive oil to ensure thorough coating
- Store in an airtight container to maintain crispiness
- Sprinkle with nutritional yeast for a cheesy flavor

Nutritional Values: Calories: 58, Fat: 3.6g, Carbs: 6g, Protein: 2g, Sugar: 0g, Sodium: 590 mg, Potassium: 213 mg, Cholesterol: 0 mg

CRISPY PARMESAN EDAMAME PODS

Preparation Time: 10 min - **Cooking Time:** 15 min - **Servings:** 4
Glycemic Index: Low(~35)
Ingredients:
- 1 lb edamame, in pods
- 1 Tbsp olive oil
- 1/4 cup Parmesan cheese, grated
- 1 tsp garlic powder
- 1/2 tsp black pepper, freshly ground
- 1/4 tsp chili flakes

Directions:

1. Preheat oven to 375°F (190°C)
2. Rinse edamame pods and pat dry
3. In a bowl, toss edamame with olive oil, garlic powder, black pepper, and chili flakes
4. Spread edamame on a baking sheet in a single layer
5. Sprinkle grated Parmesan evenly over edamame
6. Bake for 15 min until cheese is golden and edamame are crispy

Tips:
- Serve immediately for best texture
- Store any leftovers in an airtight container and reheat in the oven for crispiness

Nutritional Values: Calories: 190, Fat: 9g, Carbs: 13g, Protein: 14g, Sugar: 3g, Sodium: 150 mg, Potassium: 482 mg, Cholesterol: 4 mg

APPLE SLICES WITH ALMOND BUTTER

Preparation Time: 5 min - **Cooking Time:** none - **Servings:** 2

Glycemic Index: Low(~40)

Ingredients:

- 1 large apple, cored and sliced
- 2 Tbsp almond butter, unsweetened
- 1 tsp cinnamon, ground
- 1 tsp honey, raw
- 1 Tbsp almonds, crushed
- 1 pinch sea salt

Directions:

1. Wash, core, and slice apple into thin pieces
2. Spread unsweetened almond butter evenly over each apple slice
3. Drizzle a small amount of honey and sprinkle ground cinnamon on top of the almond butter
4. Garnish with crushed almonds and a pinch of sea salt for added flavor

Tips:

- Opt for organic apples to reduce pesticide intake
- Store almond butter at room temperature for easier spreading

Nutritional Values: Calories: 210, Fat: 11g, Carbs: 28g, Protein: 4g, Sugar: 20g, Sodium: 70 mg, Potassium: 300 mg, Cholesterol: 0 mg

CARROT STICKS WITH HUMMUS

Preparation Time: 10 min - **Cooking Time:** none - **Servings:** 2

Glycemic Index: Low(~35)

Ingredients:

- 4 large carrots, peeled and cut into sticks
- 1/2 cup hummus, homemade or store-bought
- 1 Tbsp olive oil
- 1 tsp paprika
- 1 Tbsp parsley, finely chopped
- 1 clove garlic, minced

Directions:

1. Peel and cut carrots into thin stick-like shapes
2. In a small bowl, blend hummus with olive oil, minced garlic, and paprika for a smooth, rich taste
3. Serve carrot sticks alongside the flavored hummus for dipping
4. Garnish with finely chopped parsley for a touch of freshness

Tips:

- Replace paprika with cumin for a different flavor profile
- Use lemon-infused olive oil for an additional zest

Nutritional Values: Calories: 150, Fat: 9g, Carbs: 16g, Protein: 4g, Sugar: 5g, Sodium: 210 mg, Potassium: 470 mg, Cholesterol: 0 mg

CELERY WITH COTTAGE CHEESE

Preparation Time: 5 min - **Cooking Time:** none - **Servings:** 2

Glycemic Index: Low(~30)

Ingredients:

- 4 stalks celery, washed and trimmed
- 1/2 cup cottage cheese, low-fat
- 1 Tbsp chives, chopped
- 1/2 tsp black pepper, freshly ground
- 1/4 tsp sea salt

Directions:

1. Wash and trim the celery stalks, cutting them into manageable sticks
2. Fill the concave part of each celery stalk with low-fat cottage cheese
3. Sprinkle chopped chives, black pepper, and sea salt over the cottage cheese for enhanced flavor

Tips:

- Add a dash of paprika or dill for added spice
- Chill the celery sticks before serving for a refreshing snack

Nutritional Values: Calories: 90, Fat: 2g, Carbs: 8g, Protein: 10g, Sugar: 4g, Sodium: 320 mg, Potassium: 200 mg, Cholesterol: 5 mg

BERRY AND GREEK YOGURT PARFAIT

Preparation Time: 10 min - **Cooking Time:** none - **Servings:** 2

Glycemic Index: Low(~40)

Ingredients:

- 1 cup Greek yogurt, low-fat
- 1/2 cup mixed berries (blueberries, strawberries, raspberries), fresh
- 1 Tbsp honey, raw
- 1/4 cup granola, low-sugar
- 1 tsp lemon zest

Directions:

1. In a serving glass, layer half the Greek yogurt followed by half the mixed berries
2. Drizzle some honey over the berries
3. Add another layer of Greek yogurt and the remaining berries on top

4. Finish with a sprinkle of low-sugar granola and lemon zest for a tangy flavor

Tips:
- Opt for berries with vibrant colors for the best flavor and antioxidants
- Keep the granola crunchy by adding just before serving

Nutritional Values: Calories: 230, Fat: 3g, Carbs: 36g, Protein: 14g, Sugar: 22g, Sodium: 55 mg, Potassium: 370 mg, Cholesterol: 10 mg

CUCUMBER ROLL-UPS WITH AVOCADO HUMMUS

Preparation Time: 15 min - **Cooking Time:** none - **Servings:** 4

Glycemic Index: Low(~30)

Ingredients:
- 1 large English cucumber, thinly sliced lengthwise
- 1 ripe avocado, peeled and pitted
- 1/4 cup tahini
- 2 Tbsp lime juice, fresh
- 1 garlic clove, minced
- 1/4 tsp salt
- 1/4 tsp black pepper, freshly ground
- 1/4 tsp cumin, ground
- 1/2 cup chickpeas, drained and rinsed

Directions:
1. Using a mandoline or a sharp knife, slice the cucumber into long, thin strips
2. In a food processor, combine avocado, tahini, lime juice, garlic, salt, pepper, cumin, and chickpeas and blend until smooth to create the hummus
3. Spread a thin layer of avocado hummus on each cucumber strip
4. Carefully roll up the cucumber slices and secure them with a toothpick

Tips:
- For extra spice, add a pinch of red pepper flakes to the hummus
- Store leftover hummus in an airtight container in the refrigerator

Nutritional Values: Calories: 140, Fat: 10g, Carbs: 12g, Protein: 4g, Sugar: 2g, Sodium: 200 mg, Potassium: 370 mg, Cholesterol: 0 mg

9.4. PORTABLE PROTEIN SNACKS

SAVORY TURMERIC HARD-BOILED EGGS

Preparation Time: 5 min - **Cooking Time:** 12 min - **Servings:** 4

Glycemic Index: Low(~30)

Ingredients:
- 4 large eggs

- 1 Tbsp turmeric powder
- 1 tsp black pepper, ground
- 2 tsp sea salt

Directions:

1. Place eggs in a saucepan and cover with cold water by an inch
2. Add turmeric powder, black pepper, and 1 tsp sea salt to water and stir
3. Bring to a boil over medium-high heat, then cover, turn off the heat, and let sit for 12 min
4. Transfer to cold water to stop cooking and peel once cool

Tips:
- Add a splash of vinegar to the water to facilitate peeling
- Use eggs straight from the fridge to avoid cracking during boiling

Nutritional Values: Calories: 77, Fat: 5g, Carbs: 1g, Protein: 6g, Sugar: 1g, Sodium: 629 mg, Potassium: 63 mg, Cholesterol: 186 mg

HERB-INFUSED TURKEY ROLL-UPS

Preparation Time: 10 min - **Cooking Time:** none - **Servings:** 4

Glycemic Index: Low(~40)

Ingredients:
- 8 slices turkey breast, thinly sliced
- 4 Tbsp cream cheese, reduced-fat
- 1 Tbsp chives, chopped
- 1 Tbsp dill, fresh, chopped
- 1 cucumber, peeled and cut into sticks
- 1 bell pepper, red, julienned
- Salt to taste
- Black pepper, freshly ground to taste

Directions:

1. Spread each turkey slice with cream cheese
2. Sprinkle chives and dill evenly over the cream cheese
3. Place strips of cucumber and red bell pepper at one end of the turkey slice and roll tightly
4. Season with salt and pepper to taste

Tips:
- To enhance flavor, substitute cream cheese with herbed goat cheese
- Store in a cool part of the refrigerator to maintain freshness

Nutritional Values: Calories: 135, Fat: 8g, Carbs: 3g, Protein: 12g, Sugar: 2g, Sodium: 410 mg, Potassium: 180 mg, Cholesterol: 35 mg

MIXED BERRY GREEK YOGURT CUPS

Preparation Time: 8 min - **Cooking Time:** none - **Servings:** 4

Glycemic Index: Low(~30)

Ingredients:

- 2 cups Greek yogurt, low-fat
- 1/2 cup strawberries, fresh, diced
- 1/2 cup blueberries, fresh
- 1/4 cup walnuts, chopped
- 1 Tbsp honey, natural
- 1 tsp lemon zest

Directions:

1. Mix Greek yogurt with natural honey and lemon zest in a bowl
2. Gently fold in strawberries and blueberries
3. Spoon the mixture into serving cups and top with chopped walnuts

Tips:

- Use frozen berries for a chillier snack on warm days
- Drizzle a bit more honey on top before serving for added sweetness

Nutritional Values: Calories: 150, Fat: 6g, Carbs: 18g, Protein: 10g, Sugar: 12g, Sodium: 30 mg, Potassium: 120 mg, Cholesterol: 5 mg

NO-BAKE ALMOND BUTTER PROTEIN BARS

Preparation Time: 15 min - **Cooking Time:** none - **Servings:** 8

Glycemic Index: Low(~35)

Ingredients:

- 1 cup oats, rolled, gluten-free
- 1/2 cup almond butter
- 1/4 cup honey, raw
- 1/4 cup flaxseeds, ground
- 1/4 cup chia seeds
- 1/2 cup protein powder, whey, unsweetened
- 1 tsp vanilla extract

Directions:

1. Combine oats, protein powder, flaxseeds, and chia seeds in a large bowl
2. In a separate bowl, mix almond butter, honey, and vanilla extract until smooth
3. Combine both mixtures and press firmly into a lined baking tray
4. Refrigerate for 2 hr before cutting into bars

Tips:

- Warm almond butter slightly for easier mixing

- Press mixture firmly into tray to ensure bars hold shape when cut
- Store bars in an airtight container in the fridge

Nutritional Values: Calories: 210, Fat: 12g, Carbs: 18g, Protein: 10g, Sugar: 7g, Sodium: 40 mg, Potassium: 200 mg, Cholesterol: 6 mg

SAVORY EDAMAME HUMMUS CUPS

Preparation Time: 15 min - **Cooking Time:** none - **Servings:** 4

Glycemic Index: Low(~35)

Ingredients:

- 1 C. edamame, shelled and cooked
- 2 Tbsp tahini
- 1 garlic clove, minced
- Juice of 1 lemon
- 2 Tbsp olive oil
- 1/4 tsp cumin, ground
- Salt and pepper to taste
- 4 whole-wheat pita breads, cut into quarters

Directions:

1. Blend edamame, tahini, garlic, lemon juice, olive oil, cumin, salt, and pepper in a food processor until smooth
2. Scoop the mixture into a serving bowl
3. Serve with quartered whole-wheat pita breads

Tips:

- Opt for extra virgin olive oil for a better flavor profile
- Add a sprinkle of paprika for a hint of smokiness

Nutritional Values: Calories: 210, Fat: 13g, Carbs: 17g, Protein: 9g, Sugar: 3g, Sodium: 130 mg, Potassium: 340 mg, Cholesterol: 0 mg

CHAPTER 10: INDULGENT YET HEALTHY DESSERTS

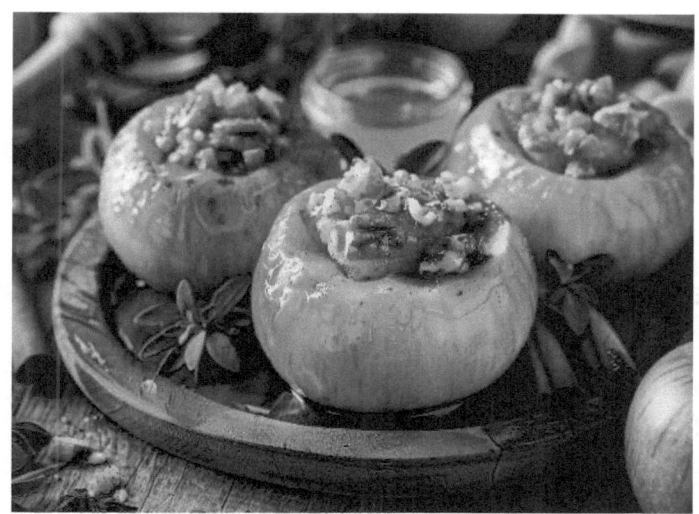

Ah, desserts! They often say that sweetness is the finale to the symphony of a good meal. Yet, when managing diabetes especially post the age of 50, indulgence in traditional sweets can feel more like a forbidden fruit than a delightful denouement. But here's a refreshing twist to the tale: desserts can indeed be both diabetic-friendly and decadent. In this chapter, we turn the tables on the misconception that desserts are off-limits, demonstrating how they can be seamlessly incorporated into your diabetic dietary regimen.

Imagine sinking your spoon into a creamy, rich pudding that tastes every bit as sinful as it looks, yet fits perfectly within your glycemic boundaries. Or picture gathering around with your grandchildren, enjoying freshly baked cookies that hold all the flavor without the worry. This isn't just wishful thinking; it's a practical reality we're going to achieve together.

The key here lies in replacing those fleeting sugar highs with hearty, healthful ingredients that enchant the palate without escalating your blood sugar. Using natural sweeteners like stevia, which impacts your blood glucose minimally, or embracing the subtle sweetness of fruits like berries and apples, you can recreate classic favorites from velvety cheesecakes to zesty lemon bars.

In crafting these recipes, we've meticulously balanced the joy of indulgence with the necessity of health management. Each recipe has been tested to assure that it not only satisfies your sweet cravings but also supports your dietary goals, maintaining that delicate balance crucial for managing diabetes effectively.

So, as we explore these sumptuous treats, remember—managing diabetes doesn't mean dessert is off the menu. It simply means rethinking and reshaping the menu to fit your life, delighting in every flavorful bite along the way. Let's rediscover the joy of desserts, transforming them from guilty pleasures to celebratory, guilt-free delights! Let the baking begin!

10.1. FRUIT-BASED DESSERTS

BAKED APPLES WITH CINNAMON

Preparation Time: 15 min - **Cooking Time:** 30 min - **Servings:** 4
Glycemic Index: Low(~38)
Ingredients:
- 4 large apples, preferably Fuji or Honeycrisp
- 1/4 C. walnuts, chopped
- 2 Tbsp raisins

- 1 Tbsp honey, raw
- 1/2 tsp cinnamon, ground
- 1/4 tsp nutmeg, ground
- 2 Tbsp butter, unsalted
- 3/4 C. water

Directions:

1. Preheat oven to 350°F (175°C)
2. Core apples and scoop out some flesh to create a well
3. Mix walnuts, raisins, honey, cinnamon, and nutmeg together
4. Stuff mixture into each apple and top each with a small dab of butter
5. Place apples in a baking dish, add water to the dish
6. Bake in preheated oven for about 30 min. or until apples are tender and stuffing is bubbly

Tips:
- Add a pinch of ground cardamom for a unique flavor twist
- Serve warm with a dollop of low-fat Greek yogurt for extra protein

Nutritional Values: Calories: 215, Fat: 9g, Carbs: 36g, Protein: 2g, Sugar: 28g, Sodium: 5 mg, Potassium: 195 mg, Cholesterol: 15 mg

GRILLED PEACHES WITH HONEY

Preparation Time: 10 min - **Cooking Time:** 12 min - **Servings:** 4

Glycemic Index: Low(~35)

Ingredients:
- 4 peaches, halved and pitted
- 1 Tbsp olive oil
- 2 Tbsp honey, raw
- 1/2 C. Greek yogurt, low-fat
- 1 Tbsp almonds, slivered
- 1/2 tsp vanilla extract

Directions:

1. Preheat grill to medium-high heat
2. Brush peach halves with olive oil
3. Grill peaches cut-side down for 6 min. until grill marks appear
4. Flip peaches and drizzle with half the honey
5. Grill for additional 6 min.
6. Serve with a dollop of Greek yogurt mixed with remaining honey and vanilla extract, sprinkle with slivered almonds

Tips:
- Consider grilling the peaches with a sprinkle of cinnamon for a spicy twist

- Pair with unsweetened iced green tea for a refreshing summer meal

Nutritional Values: Calories: 150, Fat: 4g, Carbs: 27g, Protein: 3g, Sugar: 25g, Sodium: 10 mg, Potassium: 290 mg, Cholesterol: 2 mg

BERRY COMPOTE WITH GREEK YOGURT

Preparation Time: 5 min - **Cooking Time:** 15 min - **Servings:** 4

Glycemic Index: Low(~30)

Ingredients:

- 2 C. mixed berries (blueberries, raspberries, blackberries)
- 1/4 C. water
- 2 Tbsp honey, raw
- 1 tsp lemon zest
- 1 C. Greek yogurt, low-fat

Directions:

1. Combine berries, water, honey, and lemon zest in a saucepan
2. Simmer over medium heat for about 15 min. or until berries break down into a sauce
3. Let cool slightly before serving over Greek yogurt

Tips:

- Add a sprinkle of chia seeds to the compote while cooking for added texture and nutrients
- Enhance flavor with a splash of vanilla extract during the last few minutes of simmering

Nutritional Values: Calories: 120, Fat: 1g, Carbs: 24g, Protein: 6g, Sugar: 20g, Sodium: 20 mg, Potassium: 120 mg, Cholesterol: 5 mg

MANGO SORBET

Preparation Time: 15 min - **Cooking Time:** none - **Servings:** 6

Glycemic Index: Low(~30)

Ingredients:

- 3 C. mango, fresh, cubed
- 1/4 C. lime juice
- 1/3 C. honey, raw
- 1/2 C. water
- Fresh mint leaves for garnish

Directions:

1. Puree mango, lime juice, honey, and water in a blender until smooth
2. Pour mixture into a shallow dish
3. Freeze for about 4 hr. or until firm, stirring occasionally
4. Serve garnished with fresh mint leaves

Tips:

- To enhance sweetness, adjust honey based on the ripeness of the mangoes

- Create a layered sorbet using peaches for a peach-mango twist

Nutritional Values: Calories: 110, Fat: 0g, Carbs: 28g, Protein: 1g, Sugar: 24g, Sodium: 3 mg, Potassium: 180 mg, Cholesterol: 0 mg

PAPAYA LIME SORBET

Preparation Time: 20 min - **Cooking Time:** none - **Servings:** 4

Glycemic Index: Low(~35)

Ingredients:
- 2 C. papaya, fresh and ripe, peeled and cubed
- 3 Tbsp lime juice, freshly squeezed
- 2 tsp lime zest
- ¼ C. monk fruit sweetener
- 1 tsp ginger, fresh and grated
- 1 C. water, filtered

Directions:

1. Puree papaya cubes, lime juice, lime zest, monk fruit sweetener, ginger, and water in a blender until smooth
2. Transfer the mixture to an ice cream maker and churn according to the manufacturer's instructions until it reaches a sorbet consistency
3. Transfer the sorbet to a freezer-safe container and freeze until firm, typically about 2 hr

Tips:
- To enhance the flavor, add a pinch of ground cardamom
- Serve in chilled bowls to slow down the melting process

Nutritional Values: Calories: 90, Fat: 0.1g, Carbs: 23g, Protein: 0.6g, Sugar: 12g, Sodium: 5mg, Potassium: 189mg, Cholesterol: 0mg

10.2. DIABETIC-FRIENDLY CAKES AND MUFFINS

ALMOND FLOUR BLUEBERRY MUFFINS

Preparation Time: 15 min - **Cooking Time:** 25 min - **Servings:** 12

Glycemic Index: Low(~35)

Ingredients:
- 2 cups almond flour
- 1 tsp baking soda
- ¼ tsp salt
- 3 eggs, beaten
- ¼ cup honey, raw
- 1 tsp vanilla extract
- ¼ cup unsweetened almond milk
- 1 cup blueberries, fresh

Directions:

1. Preheat oven to 350°F (177°C)
2. Grease muffin pan or line with muffin liners
3. Combine almond flour, baking soda, and salt in a large bowl
4. In another bowl, whisk together eggs, honey, vanilla extract, and almond milk
5. Add wet ingredients to dry ingredients and mix until well combined
6. Gently fold in blueberries
7. Spoon batter into prepared muffin cups, filling each about three-quarters full
8. Bake in preheated oven for 25 min or until a toothpick inserted into the center comes out clean

Tips:

- Let muffins cool for 10 min in the pan before transferring to a wire rack to cool completely
- Try using blueberries when they are in season for better flavor and nutrition

Nutritional Values: Calories: 150, Fat: 11g, Carbs: 10g, Protein: 5g, Sugar: 7g, Sodium: 130 mg, Potassium: 55 mg, Cholesterol: 55 mg

CARROT CAKE WITH CREAM CHEESE FROSTING

Preparation Time: 20 min - **Cooking Time:** 35 min - **Servings:** 8

Glycemic Index: Low(~40)

Ingredients:

- For cake: 1½ cups almond flour
- ½ cup coconut flour
- 2 tsp cinnamon, ground
- 1 tsp baking soda
- ¼ tsp salt
- 4 eggs
- ¾ cup erythritol
- ½ cup unsweetened applesauce
- ¼ cup vegetable oil
- 2 cups carrots, grated
- ½ cup walnuts, chopped | For frosting: 8 oz cream cheese, softened
- ¼ cup butter, softened
- 2 Tbsp erythritol
- 1 tsp vanilla extract

Directions:

1. Preheat oven to 350°F (177°C)
2. Grease and flour a 9-inch cake pan
3. Mix almond flour, coconut flour, cinnamon, baking soda, and salt in a bowl
4. In a separate bowl, beat eggs with erythritol, applesauce, and oil
5. Gradually add dry ingredients to wet, mixing well

6. Stir in carrots and walnuts
7. Pour batter into prepared pan
8. Bake for 35 min or until a toothpick inserted comes out clean
9. For frosting, beat cream cheese, butter, erythritol, and vanilla until smooth
10. Once cake is cool, spread frosting over the top

Tips:
- Keep cake refrigerated to maintain freshness
- Walnuts can be toasted for added flavor
- Erythritol can be substituted with another low-calorie sweetener

Nutritional Values: Calories: 320, Fat: 28g, Carbs: 15g, Protein: 7g, Sugar: 4g, Sodium: 280 mg, Potassium: 125 mg, Cholesterol: 120 mg

CHOCOLATE ZUCCHINI BREAD

Preparation Time: 15 min - **Cooking Time:** 50 min - **Servings:** 10
Glycemic Index: Low(~35)
Ingredients:
- 1½ cups almond flour
- ½ cup cocoa powder
- 1 tsp baking soda
- ¼ tsp salt
- 3 eggs
- ¼ cup unsweetened apple sauce
- ¼ cup vegetable oil
- ½ cup erythritol
- 2 cups zucchini, grated and drained
- ½ cup dark chocolate chips, sugar-free

Directions:

1. Preheat oven to 350°F (177°C)
2. Grease a 9x5 inch loaf pan
3. Mix almond flour, cocoa powder, baking soda, and salt in a large bowl
4. Beat eggs, apple sauce, oil, and erythritol in another bowl until smooth
5. Combine wet and dry ingredients, stir in zucchini and chocolate chips
6. Pour batter into prepared loaf pan
7. Bake for 50 min or until a toothpick inserted into the center comes out mostly clean

Tips:
- Let bread cool in the pan for 10 min before removing to cool completely on a wire rack
- Squeeze excess moisture from zucchini to avoid soggy bread
- Dark chocolate chips enhance the richness without added sugar

Nutritional Values: Calories: 180, Fat: 15g, Carbs: 10g, Protein: 6g, Sugar: 3g, Sodium: 220 mg, Potassium: 75 mg, Cholesterol: 55 mg

LEMON POPPY SEED MUFFINS

Preparation Time: 15 min - **Cooking Time:** 20 min - **Servings:** 12
Glycemic Index: Low(~30)
Ingredients:

- 2 cups almond flour
- 1 tsp baking soda
- ½ tsp salt
- 3 eggs
- ⅓ cup honey, raw
- ⅓ cup lemon juice, fresh
- 1 Tbsp lemon zest
- ¼ cup unsweetened almond milk
- 2 Tbsp poppy seeds

Directions:

1. Preheat oven to 375°F (190°C)
2. Grease or line a muffin tin with paper liners
3. Combine almond flour, baking soda, and salt in a large bowl
4. In another bowl, mix eggs, honey, lemon juice, lemon zest, and almond milk
5. Add wet ingredients to dry, mix until just combined
6. Fold in poppy seeds
7. Divide batter amongst muffin tins, filling each about three-quarters full
8. Bake for 20 min or until a toothpick inserted comes out clean

Tips:

- Cool muffins in the pan for 10 min before transferring to a wire rack to cool completely
- Using fresh lemon juice and zest gives a vibrant flavor
- Poppy seeds add a delightful crunch and visual appeal

Nutritional Values: Calories: 160, Fat: 12g, Carbs: 11g, Protein: 6g, Sugar: 7g, Sodium: 210 mg, Potassium: 50 mg, Cholesterol: 55 mg

SPICED PUMPKIN AND QUINOA MUFFINS

Preparation Time: 15 min - **Cooking Time:** 25 min - **Servings:** 12
Glycemic Index: Low(~45)
Ingredients:

- 1 cup quinoa flour
- 1/2 cup rolled oats
- 1/4 cup almond meal

- 1 tsp baking powder
- 1/2 tsp baking soda
- 1/4 tsp salt
- 1 tsp cinnamon, ground
- 1/2 tsp nutmeg, ground
- 1/4 tsp cloves, ground
- 1 cup pumpkin puree
- 1/4 cup olive oil
- 1/3 cup maple syrup
- 2 eggs, beaten
- 1 tsp vanilla extract
- 1/4 cup walnuts, chopped

Directions:

1. Preheat oven to 375°F (190°C)
2. In a large bowl, mix quinoa flour, oats, almond meal, baking powder, baking soda, salt, cinnamon, nutmeg, and cloves
3. In another bowl, combine pumpkin puree, olive oil, maple syrup, eggs, and vanilla extract and mix well
4. Add the wet ingredients to the dry ingredients and stir until just combined
5. Fold in chopped walnuts
6. Spoon batter into greased muffin tins and bake for 25 min. or until a toothpick comes out clean

Tips:
- Add a sprinkle of raw sugar on top before baking for a crunchy crust
- Substitute walnuts with pecans based on preference

Nutritional Values: Calories: 180, Fat: 9g, Carbs: 22g, Protein: 5g, Sugar: 7g, Sodium: 150 mg, Potassium: 134 mg, Cholesterol: 31 mg

---

10.3. HEALTHY PUDDINGS AND PARFAITS

CHIA SEED PUDDING WITH MIXED BERRIES

Preparation Time: 15 min - **Cooking Time:** none - **Servings:** 2
Glycemic Index: Low(~35)
Ingredients:
- 2 Tbsp chia seeds
- 1 C. almond milk, unsweetened
- 1/2 tsp vanilla extract
- 1 Tbsp maple syrup, sugar-free
- 1/2 C. mixed berries (blueberries, raspberries, and strawberries), fresh

- 1/4 tsp ground cinnamon

Directions:

1. Combine chia seeds, unsweetened almond milk, vanilla extract, and sugar-free maple syrup in a bowl and stir thoroughly
2. Allow the mixture to sit for 5 minutes, then stir again to prevent clumping
3. Cover and refrigerate for at least 4 hours, preferably overnight, to let the chia seeds swell
4. Serve chilled, topped with fresh mixed berries and a sprinkle of ground cinnamon

Tips:

- Opt for fresh berries for best flavor and nutrient content
- If desired, sweeten further with a stevia-based sweetener
- Stir every few hours if preparing during daytime to ensure even texture

Nutritional Values: Calories: 215, Fat: 12g, Carbs: 24g, Protein: 5g, Sugar: 8g, Sodium: 30 mg, Potassium: 201 mg, Cholesterol: 0 mg

AVOCADO CHOCOLATE PUDDING

Preparation Time: 10 min - **Cooking Time:** none - **Servings:** 2

Glycemic Index: Low(~40)

Ingredients:

- 1 ripe avocado
- 2 Tbsp cocoa powder, unsweetened
- 2 Tbsp honey, raw
- 1/4 C. Greek yogurt, plain, low-fat
- 1/2 tsp vanilla extract
- Pinch of salt

Directions:

1. Blend ripe avocado, unsweetened cocoa powder, raw honey, plain low-fat Greek yogurt, vanilla extract, and a pinch of salt in a food processor until smooth
2. Transfer the mixture to serving dishes
3. Refrigerate for at least 1 hour or until chilled

Tips:

- Serve with a dollop of whipped coconut cream for added indulgence
- Use agave syrup in place of honey for a lower glycemic alternative

Nutritional Values: Calories: 287, Fat: 19g, Carbs: 27g, Protein: 6g, Sugar: 17g, Sodium: 62 mg, Potassium: 558 mg, Cholesterol: 2 mg

Preparation Time: 15 min - **Cooking Time:** none - **Servings:** 1

Glycemic Index: Medium(~62)

Ingredients:

- 1/2 C. Greek yogurt, plain, low-fat
- 1/4 C. granola, low-sugar
- 1 Tbsp almonds, slivered
- 1/2 C. peaches, fresh, sliced
- 1 tsp honey, raw
- 1/4 tsp ground flaxseeds

Directions:

1. In a serving glass, layer half of the Greek yogurt followed by half of the granola, a few slivered almonds, and a layer of sliced fresh peaches
2. Repeat the layers once more ending with a top layer of Greek yogurt
3. Drizzle with raw honey and sprinkle ground flaxseeds on top right before serving

Tips:

- Choose firm, ripe peaches for the best flavor and texture
- Use gluten-free granola to cater to those with gluten sensitivities
- Substitute peaches with berries or mixed fruit depending on season and availability

Nutritional Values: Calories: 345, Fat: 9g, Carbs: 53g, Protein: 17g, Sugar: 28g, Sodium: 105 mg, Potassium: 412 mg, Cholesterol: 10 mg

TAPIOCA PUDDING WITH COCONUT MILK

Preparation Time: 10 min - **Cooking Time:** 20 min - **Servings:** 4

Glycemic Index: Low(~50)

Ingredients:

- 1/3 C. tapioca pearls, small
- 2 C. coconut milk, reduced-fat
- 1/3 C. xylitol
- 1 egg, beaten
- 1/2 tsp vanilla extract
- 1/4 C. shredded coconut, unsweetened
- Pinch of salt

Directions:

1. Combine reduced-fat coconut milk, xylitol, and a pinch of salt in a saucepan over medium heat until nearly boiling
2. Add small tapioca pearls and cook, stirring constantly, until the tapioca pearls become translucent and the mixture thickens, about 15 minutes

3. Remove from heat, quickly stir in beaten egg, and return to low heat for an additional 5 minutes

4. Stir in vanilla extract and unsweetened shredded coconut, then remove from heat and let cool slightly before serving

Tips:

- Serve warm for creamy texture
- Sprinkle cinnamon or nutmeg on top before serving for added spice
- Store leftovers in the fridge and enjoy cold as a refreshing treat

Nutritional Values: Calories: 230, Fat: 9g, Carbs: 36g, Protein: 3g, Sugar: 1g, Sodium: 30 mg, Potassium: 210 mg, Cholesterol: 32 mg

ROASTED PEACH AND THYME PUDDING

Preparation Time: 15 min - **Cooking Time:** 45 min - **Servings:** 4
Glycemic Index: Low(~35)
Ingredients:

- 3 medium peaches, pitted and halved
- 2 tsp fresh thyme, finely chopped
- 1 C. almond flour
- ¼ C. erythritol
- 1 egg, beaten
- 1 tsp vanilla extract
- ½ C. almond milk, unsweetened
- 1 tsp baking powder
- ¼ tsp salt

Directions:

1. Preheat oven to 375°F (190°C)
2. Place peach halves cut-side up in a baking dish and sprinkle with half the thyme
3. In a mixing bowl, combine almond flour, erythritol, baking powder, and salt
4. In another bowl, mix almond milk, egg, and vanilla extract
5. Combine wet and dry ingredients until smooth and pour over peaches
6. Sprinkle remaining thyme on top
7. Bake for 45 min or until golden and set

Tips:

- Serve warm with a dollop of Greek yogurt if desired
- Adding a pinch of nutmeg can enhance the thyme's aromatic nature
- Opt for ripe but firm peaches to maintain structure during baking

Nutritional Values: Calories: 180, Fat: 12g, Carbs: 15g, Protein: 5g, Sugar: 8g, Sodium: 150 mg, Potassium: 200 mg, Cholesterol: 53 mg

OATMEAL AND RAISIN COOKIES

Preparation Time: 15 min - **Cooking Time:** 10 min - **Servings:** 12

Glycemic Index: Low(~55)

Ingredients:

- 1½ C. rolled oats
- ¾ C. whole wheat flour
- ½ tsp baking soda
- ¼ tsp salt
- ¼ C. coconut oil, melted
- ½ C. agave nectar
- 1 large egg, beaten
- ½ tsp vanilla extract
- ½ C. raisins

Directions:

1. Preheat oven to 350°F (175°C)
2. In a large bowl, combine rolled oats, whole wheat flour, baking soda, and salt
3. In another bowl, whisk together melted coconut oil, agave nectar, beaten egg, and vanilla extract
4. Mix wet ingredients into dry ingredients until well combined
5. Fold in raisins
6. Drop tablespoon-sized portions onto a baking sheet lined with parchment paper
7. Bake for 10 min or until edges are golden brown

Tips:

- Let cookies cool on the baking sheet for 5 min before transferring to a wire rack to cool completely
- Store in an airtight container to maintain freshness

Nutritional Values: Calories: 130, Fat: 5g, Carbs: 20g, Protein: 2g, Sugar: 9g, Sodium: 80 mg, Potassium: 75 mg, Cholesterol: 15 mg

ALMOND BUTTER COOKIES

Preparation Time: 12 min - **Cooking Time:** 8 min - **Servings:** 15

Glycemic Index: Low(~50)

Ingredients:

- 1 C. almond butter
- 1/3 C. honey, raw
- 1 egg
- ½ tsp baking soda

- ¼ tsp salt
- ½ C. dark chocolate chips, sugar-free

Directions:

1. Preheat oven to 375°F (190°C)
2. In a bowl, mix almond butter, raw honey, and egg until smooth
3. Stir in baking soda and salt
4. Add sugar-free dark chocolate chips and stir until evenly distributed
5. Drop by teaspoonfuls onto a parchment-lined baking sheet
6. Bake for 8 min or until the edges begin to turn brown

Tips:

- Cookies will be soft initially; they harden as they cool
- For a nuttier flavor, add a sprinkle of ground flaxseeds before baking

Nutritional Values: Calories: 160, Fat: 12g, Carbs: 10g, Protein: 5g, Sugar: 7g, Sodium: 100 mg, Potassium: 150 mg, Cholesterol: 20 mg

COCONUT FLOUR BROWNIES

Preparation Time: 15 min - **Cooking Time:** 20 min - **Servings:** 8
Glycemic Index: Low(~45)
Ingredients:

- ¾ C. coconut flour
- ½ C. unsweetened cocoa powder
- ¼ tsp salt
- ½ C. coconut oil, melted
- ¼ C. honey
- 1 tsp vanilla extract
- 3 eggs

Directions:

1. Preheat oven to 350°F (175°C)
2. In a bowl, mix together coconut flour, cocoa powder, and salt
3. In another bowl, combine melted coconut oil, honey, vanilla extract, and eggs
4. Add wet ingredients to dry ingredients and stir until well combined
5. Pour batter into an 8x8 inch (20x20 cm) baking dish lined with parchment paper
6. Smooth the top with a spatula
7. Bake for 20 min or until a toothpick inserted into the center comes out clean

Tips:

- Cool in the dish for 10 min, then lift out using the parchment and cut into squares
- Dust with additional cocoa powder for a richer taste

Nutritional Values: Calories: 180, Fat: 14g, Carbs: 12g, Protein: 4g, Sugar: 7g, Sodium: 75 mg, Potassium: 90 mg, Cholesterol: 70 mg

NO-BAKE GRANOLA BARS

Preparation Time: 20 min - **Cooking Time:** none - **Servings:** 10

Glycemic Index: Low(~48)

Ingredients:

- 1 C. rolled oats
- ¼ C. flaxseed, ground
- ½ C. almond butter
- ¼ C. honey, raw
- ½ C. dried cranberries
- ¼ C. sunflower seeds, unsalted
- 1 tsp cinnamon, ground

Directions:

1. Combine rolled oats, ground flaxseed, dried cranberries, unsalted sunflower seeds, and ground cinnamon in a large bowl
2. In a small saucepan over low heat, warm almond butter and raw honey until smooth and well combined
3. Pour the almond butter mixture over the dry ingredients and stir until everything is sticky and evenly coated
4. Press mixture firmly into a lined 8x8 inch (20x20 cm) baking pan
5. Chill in the refrigerator for at least 2 hrs before cutting into bars

Tips:

- Cut bars when fully chilled to maintain shape
- Wrap bars individually for an easy grab-and-go snack

Nutritional Values: Calories: 195, Fat: 10g, Carbs: 23g, Protein: 5g, Sugar: 12g, Sodium: 15 mg, Potassium: 175 mg, Cholesterol: 0 mg

SPICED CARROT AND QUINOA BARS

Preparation Time: 15 min - **Cooking Time:** 25 min - **Servings:** 12

Glycemic Index: Low(~45)

Ingredients:

- 1 cup quinoa flakes
- 1 cup almond flour
- ½ cup unsweetened applesauce
- ¼ cup coconut oil, melted
- 2 Tbsp ground flaxseed mixed with 6 Tbsp water
- ¾ cup carrots, grated

- 1 tsp cinnamon
- ½ tsp nutmeg
- ¼ tsp ground ginger
- 1 tsp baking powder
- 1 pinch of salt

Directions:

1. Preheat oven to 350°F (175°C)
2. In a large bowl, combine quinoa flakes, almond flour, cinnamon, nutmeg, ginger, baking powder, and salt
3. In a separate bowl, whisk together flaxseed mixture, applesauce, and melted coconut oil
4. Combine wet and dry ingredients, then fold in grated carrots
5. Spread mixture evenly in a greased 9x9 inch baking pan
6. Bake for 25 min or until the edges start to turn golden brown and a toothpick inserted into the center comes out clean
7. Let cool before slicing into bars

Tips:

- Store bars in an airtight container to maintain freshness
- Add a sprinkle of chopped walnuts or pecans for extra texture and flavor

Nutritional Values: Calories: 160, Fat: 9g, Carbs: 18g, Protein: 4g, Sugar: 2g, Sodium: 75 mg, Potassium: 135 mg, Cholesterol: 0 mg

PART IV: ENHANCING YOUR LIFESTYLE

CHAPTER 11. INCORPORATING EXERCISE AND PHYSICAL ACTIVITY

Imagine stepping out into the early morning light, the air crisp and expectant, as you set forth on a gentle walk. This simple act, often overlooked in the hustle of our daily routines, is more than just a form of physical exercise; it's a profound demonstration of your commitment to enhancing your lifestyle in your golden years.

As we navigate the intricacies of managing diabetes after 50, incorporating consistent physical activity into our days emerges as a cornerstone—not just for its well-documented health benefits but as an enriching element of daily life. Exercise in our mature years does wonders, extending beyond the realm of physical health benefits to mental clarity and emotional stability.

Why, you might ask, is exercise so crucial, especially for those of us managing diabetes? Engaging in physical activity helps to regulate blood sugar levels and increases insulin sensitivity, meaning that your body becomes better at handling the sugars you ingest without sudden spikes or ominous plummets. But the magic of movement extends its tendrils further into the fabric of our mental health, helping to dissipate stress, elevate our mood, and sharpen our minds against the fog that can sometimes descend in later years.

You don't need to morph into an athlete overnight, nor should you. The beauty of integrating exercise into your life at this stage is the vast array of options that fit varying levels of ability and interest. Whether it's swimming, gardening, yoga, or brisk walking, the aim is to find activities that not only manage your blood sugar but also bring joy and revitalization.

Let this chapter serve as your guide to weaving exercise seamlessly into your lifestyle, with adaptable strategies that respect your body's limits while challenging it to regain and maintain strength and vitality. We'll explore not just the "how" but the invigorating "why" of staying active, ensuring that each step you take is grounded in a desire to live fully and healthily. Here, we pair inspiration with practical advice, setting you on a path to discovering the most enjoyable and beneficial forms of exercise tailored specifically to your life's rich tapestry.

11.1 WHY EXERCISE IS CRUCIAL: BENEFITS BEYOND WEIGHT LOSS

Engaging in regular physical activity is one of those universal recommendations that spans across various health advisories – akin to eating your vegetables or ensuring you get enough sleep. But as adults over fifty managing diabetes, the call for physical activity rings with a different urgency and a plethora of tailored benefits that go beyond mere weight loss. It's not only about shedding pounds or maintaining a trim waistline; exercise plays multiple, crucial roles in your holistic health landscape.

Firstly, at its core, physical activity helps control blood glucose levels. When you exercise, your muscles demand energy derived from glucose in the bloodstream, which helps lower blood sugar levels naturally. This process is crucial for managing diabetes, as it supplements your dietary efforts to regulate these levels. Moreover, regular exercise improves insulin sensitivity, which means less insulin is required to manage blood sugar levels, a truly beneficial cycle.

But let's dive deeper and explore how regular physical activity benefits us profoundly, echoing well beyond these immediate effects. As we embed movement into our daily routines, we start a positive domino effect that can lead to improved heart health, enhanced mental well-being, and a fortified defense against a host of diabetes-related complications.

Protecting Your Heart

Heart disease is a significant risk for those with diabetes, with the condition causing changes to the blood vessels and heart. Regular physical activity strengthens the heart muscle, improves blood flow, and increases heart efficiency. It's like giving your heart the workout it needs to stay strong and efficient. Activities such as brisk walking, cycling, or swimming, elevate the heart rate, which can help reduce arterial stiffness and lower blood pressure, mitigating one of the significant risk factors associated with heart complications.

Enhancing Mental Well-being

The benefits of exercise aren't confined to our physical health. Engaging in regular physical activity is also a pivotal strategy in managing psychological wellbeing. Exercise is associated with the release of endorphins, often dubbed 'feel-good' hormones, which can lift mood naturally. For individuals managing chronic conditions like diabetes, this is especially relevant as mental health challenges such as depression and anxiety can occur at higher rates.

Regular exercise also offers a profound counter to stress. Stress, particularly chronic stress, can have deleterious effects on blood sugar levels, due to the release of stress hormones like cortisol and adrenaline, which can spike blood sugar. Participating in physical activities provides a release valve for stress, assisting in managing these hormonal levels and promoting a calmer, more balanced state of mind.

Combating Neuropathy and Enhancing Mobility

Diabetic neuropathy is a type of nerve damage that can occur in people with diabetes. Symptoms include numbness, tingling, pain, or weakness in the feet and hands. Regular activity promotes blood flow to the limbs, which helps to nourish damaged nerves and keep them functioning as optimally as possible. Furthermore, maintaining a regimen of regular movement can help prevent common diabetic complications like foot ulcers by promoting better circulation.

As mobility can potentially decrease with age, staying active ensures that joints remain flexible, muscles are strong, and balance is maintained. These benefits are crucial in preventing falls, a common cause of serious injury in older adults.

Aiding Digestive Health

Exercise also encourages a healthy digestive tract. Regular movement helps to boost metabolism and can aid in maintaining a healthy weight, reducing the strain on your digestive system and helping to regulate appetite. This can be particularly beneficial as medications for diabetes, and the condition itself can sometimes disturb normal digestive processes, leading to issues like gastroparesis.

Promoting Longevity and Quality of Life

Living with diabetes can feel overwhelming at times. Incorporating exercise into your routine can lead to improved sleep patterns, better energy levels, and an overall enhanced quality of life. Exercise can extend life expectancy not only by reducing the risks associated with diabetes but by improving holistic health in general.

Building Social Connections

Exercising, especially in group settings such as classes, walking groups, or community events, can also have the added benefit of enhancing your social connections. Engaging with others in healthy activities can provide emotional support, reduce feelings of isolation, and boost your motivation to stay active.

Regular physical activity transcends the basic need for physical health; it weaves into the fabric of your mental, emotional, and social well-being, presenting a cornerstone in the management of diabetes after 50. It empowers not only your body but your spirit, reinforcing your resilience against complications, enhancing your enjoyment of life, and elevating your overall health trajectory.

As we delve deeper into specific types of exercises and practical tips in the following sections, remember: the journey of a thousand miles begins with a single step. Let this be your step towards not just managing, but thriving with diabetes in your enriching later years.

11.2 CUSTOMIZED WORKOUTS FOR THOSE OVER 50

Navigating the landscape of exercise can seem daunting as we age, especially when managing a condition like diabetes. The body isn't as forgiving as it once was, and concerns about injury or overexertion are valid. However, this shouldn't deter us from activity; instead, it calls for a more tailored, thoughtful approach to exercise that respects the unique needs of those over 50 with diabetes.

Embracing physical activity at this stage of life means understanding that one size does not fit all. Customized workout plans that cater to individual health status, fitness levels, and personal preferences are not just beneficial—they are essential for sustainable, enjoyable, and effective physical activity.

Understanding the Starting Point

The journey into customized workouts begins with a clear understanding of one's current health status. This involves consulting with healthcare providers to assess how diabetes and other age-related factors like bone density, joint health, cardiovascular status, and overall physical fitness might influence exercise choices. These initial evaluations provide the groundwork, ensuring that the activities chosen enhance health without risking harm.

Developing Tailored Workout Regimens

Each individual's workout plan should reflect not only medical advisories but personal interests and lifestyle. Here's how we can approach this:

1. Mixing Cardiovascular and Strength Training

A balanced approach that incorporates both aerobic (cardiovascular) and anaerobic (strength training) exercises can optimize health benefits. Cardio exercises like walking, swimming, or cycling help improve heart health and manage weight, crucial for controlling diabetes. On the other hand, strength training with light weights or resistance bands can help build muscle mass, which is vital as muscle tissue helps in the efficient absorption and utilization of glucose from the bloodstream.

2. Incorporating Flexibility and Balance Exercises

As we age, maintaining flexibility and balance becomes just as important as building strength and endurance. Exercises like yoga or Tai Chi not only enhance flexibility and balance but also reduce stress and improve mental health. These activities are low-impact and can be easily adapted to different fitness levels and physical limitations.

3. Interval Training Adaptations

High-Intensity Interval Training (HIIT) might sound intimidating, but it can be adjusted for those over 50. Modified HIIT, involving short bursts of moderate activity followed by rest periods, can be a highly effective way to improve cardiovascular and metabolic health without the strain of prolonged high-intensity exercise.

Staying Safe and Preventing Injuries

Customization also means prioritizing safety to prevent injuries. This involves:

- **Warm-ups and Cool-downs**: Starting workouts with gentle stretching and gradually increasing the intensity prepares the body for activity and reduces the risk of injuries. Similarly, ending sessions with cool-down exercises and stretches helps in muscle recovery and reduces post-exercise soreness.
- **Hydration and Blood Sugar Management**: Staying hydrated is crucial, especially since dehydration can impact blood sugar levels. Monitoring blood sugar before, during, and after exercise can prevent undesirable spikes or dangerous drops, ensuring that adjustments to activity levels or meal plans can be made promptly.

Listening to the Body

One of the most critical aspects of a customized workout plan is learning to listen to one's body. Recognizing the signs of too much exertion or when an exercise does not feel right is crucial. Adjustments should be made based on feedback from the body—this might mean altering the intensity, duration, or even the form of exercise.

Regular Reviews and Adjustments

Finally, a customized workout regimen is not static. Regular reviews with healthcare professionals ensure that as health changes—whether improvements from regular activity or new challenges that arise with aging—workout plans evolve too. This might mean increasing intensity, trying new activities, or sometimes, pulling back when necessary.

Through a customized approach, exercise becomes not just a directive but a personally molded lifestyle choice, enhancing both physical and psychological wellbeing. By tailoring activities to individual needs, capabilities, and enjoyment, those over 50 with diabetes can transform their relationship with exercise from a medical must to a cherished part of daily life, reaping benefits that radiate through all aspects of health.

11.3 PRACTICAL TIPS FOR STAYING ACTIVE

Staying active in later years, especially while managing diabetes, calls for more than casual recommendations; it demands practical, achievable, and motivating strategies that integrate naturally into your lifestyle. Let's explore how small, actionable steps can encourage a habit of activity, weaving these into the fabric and rhythm of daily life.

The foundation of staying active revolves not just around formal regimens but incorporating movement throughout your day. This blended approach helps maintain blood sugar levels consistently and leverages opportunities for exercise that you might not have considered.

Embed Movement in Daily Routines

Transform your daily routines into opportunities for activity. Practicing this consistently turns mundane tasks into beneficial physical exertions. Consider parking further away from store entrances, opting for stairs instead of elevators, and if feasible, using a stand-up desk or taking five-minute movement breaks each hour during sedentary activities. These small integrations can significantly enhance your daily activity level without feeling like a burden.

Set Realistic Goals

Establish clear, achievable goals. Perhaps start with walking 10 minutes per day, then gradually increase the duration and intensity as your stamina and health improve. These goals should feel challenging yet achievable, tailored to your current fitness level and health conditions. Celebrating these small victories can provide a significant psychological boost.

Use Technology Wisely

Technology offers incredible tools for boosting activity levels. Pedometers, fitness trackers, and smartphone apps not only help monitor your daily activity levels but also set reminders to move or track your progress against your goals. These devices can serve as a motivator and a digital companion in your journey towards consistent physical activity.

Create a Weekly Schedule

Planning is crucial. Outline your weekly physical activities, integrating variety to keep things interesting. Maybe it's swimming on Monday, a gentle yoga class on Wednesday, and a walk in the park on Friday. This not only aids in establishing a routine but also ensures a balanced approach that covers cardiovascular, strength, and flexibility training.

Join Groups or Classes

There is significant power in community. Joining exercise groups or classes can provide social encouragement and motivation. Whether it's a dance class geared towards older adults or a walking group, these gatherings can offer support and structure. Plus, they make physical activity a social and enjoyable event which can help sustain long-term commitment.

Understand Your Body's Feedback

Listening to your body is non-negotiable. Recognize signs of overexertion, such as undue pain, heavy breathlessness, or extreme fatigue. Adjusting your activity level in response to your body's messages is critical to avoid injury and maintain a positive relationship with exercise.

Stay Flexible with Indoor Options

Weather or other external conditions can disrupt the best-laid plans. Have a backup plan for indoor activities so that your physical activity doesn't falter when it's too rainy for a walk or too hot for a bike ride. Simple indoor exercises, like stair climbing, practicing yoga, or workout videos, can be excellent alternatives.

Consult and Coordinate with Healthcare Providers

Maintain open communication with your healthcare team about your exercise plans and experiences. They can offer guidance tailored to your health status, adjusting recommendations as your fitness level or health conditions change. This healthcare provider can act as a safeguard and a guide in optimizing your exercise regimen.

Incorporate Mindfulness and Meditation

While meditation itself isn't a physical exercise, it contributes significantly to mental health and overall well-being, which are essential for sustaining an active lifestyle. Mindfulness practices can enhance your awareness of the body's needs and responses to different physical activities, fostering a deeper connection and appreciation for your body's capabilities.

Keep It Fun and Enjoyable

Finally, ensure that whatever activity you choose, it brings you joy. The pleasure derived from activity boosts adherence. Whether it's the meditative rhythm of swimming laps, the exhilarating rush of a dance class, or the tranquil pleasure of a morning walk, finding joy in these activities will keep you motivated.

By weaving these practical strategies into your daily life, you ensure that staying active after 50 is not just a doctor's directive but a fulfilling, integral part of your daily existence. These strategies acknowledge the limitations and opportunities of aging, tailoring exercise to enhance your lifestyle, not just extend it. Through thoughtful, personalized, and enjoyable activities, you can look forward to each day with vitality and enthusiasm, making well-being an accessible and delightful reality.

CHAPTER 12. EMOTIONAL AND MENTAL HEALTH

When we talk about diabetes management, particularly after reaching the milestone age of 50, our focus often tends to lean heavily on the physical—what to eat, how much to exercise, and managing blood sugar levels. Yet, there's a vital component of our well-being that sometimes drifts into the shadows, unspoken yet profoundly impactful: our emotional and mental health.

Navigating life with diabetes can stir a cocktail of emotions—frustration, anxiety, and even bouts of depression. These feelings can sneak up subtly, dimming the vibrant life you're meant to live. But just as we adopt dietary changes and physical routines, attending to our mental landscape is equally crucial. It's about shifting the lens, not just to survive with diabetes but to thrive with it.

Imagine this: You've had a challenging day; blood sugar levels aren't cooperating despite your best efforts. The frustration bubbles. Here, cultivating mental resilience isn't just helpful; it's essential. It's about building a toolkit to manage stress, an unwavering ally as immediate and supportive as a comforting meal or a walk in your favorite park.

The power of resilience shines through in not just bouncing back but in stepping forward with confidence and a smile. It involves embracing techniques of mindfulness, perhaps a gentle delve into meditation, or the simple act of breathing deeply, consciously. These methods aren't merely escapes but bridges to a stronger, more serene you.

But let's not tread this path solemnly. Laughter, joy, connection—these are not just permissible; they are prescriptions for a well-rounded life. Engaging with friends, sharing your challenges, and yes, laughing over the quirks of life even when it seems to hand you lemons, are pivotal.

In this chapter, we don't just acknowledge the emotional rollercoaster that can accompany diabetes; we embrace it, we equip ourselves for it, and crucially, we learn not to journey through it alone—because mental health, much like a diet, benefits profoundly from a balanced, well-nourished approach. The goal? To ensure you're not just managing diabetes but living fully, richly, and vibrantly, beyond the numbers on a glucose meter.

12.1 MANAGING STRESS, ANXIETY, AND DEPRESSION

Managing stress, anxiety, and depression as someone over 50 with diabetes isn't just a sideline to your physical health regime—it's as critical as monitoring your blood glucose or planning your meals. Many find the emotional terrain of living with a chronic condition like diabetes to be challenging and at times, overwhelming. However, within these challenges lies an opportunity to harness resilience, reduce distress, and enhance your overall well-being.

Imagine, for a moment, the intricate dance of managing a health condition that requires constant attention. One might say it's akin to balancing on a tightrope while juggling—where each ball represents different aspects of your life, such as family responsibilities, personal interests, and, of course, health management. This balancing act is made considerably tougher by stress, anxiety, and bouts of depression, which can feel like gusts of wind threatening to throw you off balance.

Stress, particularly, can be a stealthy saboteur. It can elevate blood sugar levels indirectly by triggering the release of stress hormones like cortisol and adrenaline. These hormones kick your liver into high gear, releasing stored glucose to boost energy. But for someone with diabetes, this well-intended surge can tip the scales, leading to higher glucose levels. Reducing stress isn't merely relaxing—it's a direct contributor to stabilizing glucose levels.

The story of anxiety intertwines closely with stress but adds its unique twist. It's that persistent concern about the 'what ifs'—what if my blood sugar drops? What if I have a diabetic emergency while alone? Unlike stress, anxiety is less about what's happening right now and more about anticipating what could go wrong. Yet, the physiological response can be similar, with your body releasing hormones that might interfere with your well-being.

Depression casts a longer, often more debilitating shadow. It can sap your motivation and energy, making diabetes management feel not just challenging, but insurmountable. Depression isn't just a bad day; it's a pervasive feeling of emptiness or despair that holds on and doesn't let go easily.

Dealing with these emotional states starts by recognizing their presence and understanding that it's not just 'all in your head.' These are genuine biological and psychological responses that can affect your physical health. Let's explore some strategies to manage these feelings effectively:

Transforming Stress with Techniques That Actually Work

First, identify the stressors. What specific aspects of diabetes management, or life more generally, trigger stress? Once you know your triggers, you can work on practical methods to mitigate them. Techniques like mindfulness and meditation can be profoundly effective. Mindfulness teaches you to stay present, focused, and grounded, reducing the overwhelm of past regrets and future anxieties. There's also a place for structured relaxation techniques such as progressive muscle relaxation or deep breathing exercises. These can be particularly useful during moments of acute stress, helping to calm the body's physiological response and offering a refreshing mental reset.

The Anxiety-Alleviation Game Plan

For anxiety, cognitive-behavioral strategies are a powerhouse. Techniques like cognitive reframing allow you to challenge and change the fearful thoughts that fuel anxiety. Instead of thinking, "What if I have a hypoglycemic episode while I'm out?", reframe it to, "I am prepared to manage my blood sugar levels effectively, and I know how to get help if I need it."

Regular physical activity is another linchpin in managing anxiety. Exercise releases endorphins—often referred to as feel-good hormones—while simultaneously burning away stress hormone accumulations. Moreover, routine exercise can strengthen your confidence in your body's health and resilience, a direct counter to anxiety's whispers of doubt.

Combatting Depression with Regiment and Support

When it comes to battling depression, routine and support are your allies. Establish a daily routine that incorporates not just necessary tasks but meaningful and enjoyable activities—be it gardening, reading, or other hobbies that light a spark in your day.

Don't underestimate the power of social support. Stay connected with family, friends, or support groups where you can share experiences and challenges. Sometimes, just knowing that there are others who understand what you're going through can lighten the emotional load substantially.

In some cases, therapy may be a critical part of managing depression. Therapists can provide tailored strategies to cope with feelings, work through emotional baggage, and set realistic, attainable goals.

Integrating Nutritional Well-being with Emotional Resilience

Lastly, while this isn't a chapter about specific recipes, recognize that what you eat can influence how you feel. A well-balanced diet that stabilizes blood sugar levels within the target range can also stabilize your mood. Omega-3 fatty acids, found in fish and flaxseeds, are known for their mood-boosting properties. Meanwhile, complex carbohydrates are excellent for a slow release of glucose into the bloodstream, which can keep your mood steady.

In closing, managing stress, anxiety, and depression requires a dedicated approach influenced by both psychological and physical practices. The journey of managing diabetes is not just about the body; it encompasses the complex, beautiful weave of body, mind, and spirit. By addressing each aspect with care and detailed attention, you empower yourself to lead not just a healthy life, but a happy and fulfilled one.

12.2 BUILDING RESILIENCE AND MAINTAINING A POSITIVE OUTLOOK

Resilience and a positive outlook may seem like qualities bestowed at birth, inherent traits that some are lucky to possess. Yet, these are skills, much like preparing a gourmet meal or mastering an exercise routine. They can be learned, honed, and mastered, especially when managing a condition like diabetes after 50, a time when life's challenges could easily tilt towards the overwhelming.

Building resilience in the face of diabetes is akin to constructing a house, brick by brick, with each brick representing a strategy, a habit, or a mindset shift. Over time, these elements create a robust structure that shelters you from the metaphorical storms of health worries and emotional disturbances.

The Foundation of Resilience: Understanding and Acceptance

Start by laying a strong foundation with understanding and acceptance—understanding your condition and accepting that while diabetes is a part of your life, it does not define your entire existence. This acceptance doesn't mean resignation but rather, acknowledging the reality, which is the first step towards empowerment.

The Walls: Healthy Routines and Self-Care

Build the walls of your resilience house with routines that promote physical health and emotional well-being. Establish a daily regimen that includes monitoring your blood sugar, preparing nutritious meals, and engaging in physical activity. But self-care extends beyond physical care; it also involves giving yourself permission to rest, to enjoy hobbies, and to connect with loved ones. These activities nourish the soul and fortify the mind.

The Roof: Social Support

No house is complete without a roof, and in the architecture of resilience, this roof is social support. The connections you forge with family, friends, and support groups provide shelter from the adversities of life. They offer not just emotional comfort but practical assistance and a sharing of experiences that reminds you, you're not navigating this path alone.

Windows and Doors: Mindfulness and Openness to Experience

Incorporate windows and doors into your resilience home through mindfulness and an openness to new experiences. Mindfulness keeps you centered and present, helping manage the stress and anxiety that often accompany chronic conditions like diabetes. Openness leads you to new information, perspectives, and potentially beneficial experiences, such as meditation classes, dietary workshops, or even new technologies for diabetes management.

Decorating Your Resilient Home: Positive Thinking

Adorn your resilient home with the decor of positive thinking. This isn't about ignoring reality or painting challenges with a rosy hue. Instead, it involves focusing on the strengths you have, the progress you make, and the small victories along the way. It's about reframing setbacks as opportunities to learn and grow.

Regular Maintenance: Continuous Learning and Adaptation

Just as a house requires ongoing maintenance, so does your resilience. Stay informed about the latest in diabetes care, continue to adapt your diet and exercise routines as needed, and remain flexible in your approach to challenges. Resilience is not static but dynamically evolves as your circumstances change.

Gardens and Surroundings: Cultivating Interests and Engaging with Life

Finally, do not forget the gardens and surroundings of your resilience home. Cultivate interests outside of diabetes management. Whether it's gardening, painting, writing, or volunteering, engaging in activities that fulfill you can enhance your sense of purpose and well-being. These pursuits provide a buffer against stress and enrich your quality of life.

Building resilience and maintaining a positive outlook is a journey that involves more than just managing your diabetes—it requires managing your life in a holistic and harmonious way. The resilience you build helps you not only to cope with diabetes but also to thrive despite it.

Remember, the house of resilience isn't built in a day. Each small step you take is a brick added to your structure. Each day you choose to reach out for support, indulge in self-care, learn something new, or shift a negative thought pattern is a day you build stronger walls, a sturdier roof, and a more joyful living space within yourself.

Through the construction of this resilient home, you pave a path towards not just living, but thriving. You redefine what it means to live with diabetes. With every brick of resilience, every sweep of positive paint, you transform challenges into stepping stones and prove that life's second act can be its most definitive.

MEASUREMENT CONVERSION TABLE

Volume Measurements

US Measurement	Metric Measurement
1 tsp (tsp)	5 milliliters (ml)
1 tbsp (tbsp)	15 milliliters (ml)
1 fluid ounce (fl oz)	30 milliliters (ml)
1 Cup	240 milliliters (ml)
1 pint (2 Cs)	470 milliliters (ml)
1 quart (4 Cs)	0.95 liters (L)
1 gallon (16 Cs)	3.8 liters (L)

Weight Measurements

US Measurement	Metric Measurement
1 ounce (oz)	28 grams (g)
1 pound (lb)	450 grams (g)
1 pound (lb)	0.45 kilograms (kg)

Length Measurements

US Measurement	Metric Measurement
1 inch (in)	2.54 centimeters (cm)
1 foot (ft)	30.48 centimeters (cm)
1 foot (ft)	0.3048 meters (m)
1 yard (yd)	0.9144 meters (m)

Temperature Conversions

Fahrenheit (°F)	Celsius (°C)
32°F	0°C
212°F	100°C
Formula: (°F - 32) x 0.5556 = °C	Formula: (°C x 1.8) + 32 = °F

Oven Temperature Conversions

US Oven Term	Fahrenheit (°F)	Celsius (°C)
Very Slow	250°F	120°C
Slow	300-325°F	150-165°C
Moderate	350-375°F	175-190°C
Moderately Hot	400°F	200°C
Hot	425-450°F	220-230°C
Very Hot	475-500°F	245-260°C

BONUS:

15 Air Fryer Recipes

THANK YOU FOR YOUR PURCHASE!

Dear Reader,

Thank you so much for purchasing my book! I truly hope it provides you with value and enjoyment. Your support plays a crucial role in my journey as an author and is deeply appreciated.

If you could spare a few moments to leave a review, I would be incredibly grateful. Your insights help me to improve and aid others in discovering books that match their interests.

Also, as a special thank you, I've included a QR code below. Please scan it to access exclusive bonus content crafted just for you.

Warm regards,

Emil Gunner

CONCLUSION

• CONTINUING YOUR HEALTH JOURNEY: NEXT STEPS

As you turn the pages of this journey—one laden with challenges and triumphs alike—you may find yourself at a poignant crossroads. Here, the initial blueprint fades and the continuous path of managing diabetes in your golden years begins. This isn't the end; rather, it's a vibrant new chapter in your personal saga of health and fulfillment.

Understanding that every step you've taken so far has been instrumental, you might now wonder, "What comes next?" The truth is, the journey continues and evolves, just as we do. Today, let's explore how you can maintain and even enhance your strides towards better health and a more joyful life.

Unfolding the Map of Tomorrow

Imagine your health journey as an ever-expanding map. Each discipline and knowledge you've acquired is a marker. But beyond the edges of this map lie uncharted territories and new discoveries. Your commitment to managing diabetes doesn't stop as you reach a milestone; it grows and adapts with time.

Embrace Lifelong Learning

Your education about diabetes should not stagnate. The scientific and medical communities are constantly uncovering new findings about dietary impacts on blood sugar, the effectiveness of exercise routines, and even the psychology of chronic illness management. Stay curious and informed:

- Subscribe to reputable health newsletters.
- Attend workshops or webinars.
- Join community groups with a focus on diabetic health.

This continuous learning will not only empower you but also invigorate your daily routine with fresh ideas and methodologies.

Refining Your Diet Over Time

While the recipes and meal plans provided have set a foundation, your dietary needs may evolve. Metabolism changes with age, and what works today might need adjustment tomorrow. Listen to your body's cues. If certain foods start to affect you differently, consider revisiting your dietician or nutritionist to refine your meal plan. This adaptation process is not a setback but a normal part of managing a dynamic condition like diabetes.

Advanced Monitoring Techniques

As technology advances, so do the tools available for diabetes management. Continuous glucose monitoring systems and smart insulin pumps are becoming more mainstream and might offer a way to get detailed insights into your glucose levels and how they fluctuate during the day. Discuss these options with your healthcare provider to determine if they could enhance your control over your condition.

The Physical Dimension: Exercise and Beyond

Physical activity remains a cornerstone of diabetes management, especially after 50. The key is to find activities that you enjoy and can sustain long term. Whether it's yoga, swimming, or simply walking, the best exercise is the one you keep doing. Moreover, consider seasonal variations or joining classes that specifically cater to your age group, keeping it both social and stimulating.

Cultivating Mindfulness and Resilience

The psychological aspects of living with diabetes often get less attention, yet they are just as crucial. Cultivating a practice of mindfulness can enhance your emotional well-being. Techniques such as meditation, deep-breathing exercises, or journaling can mitigate stress and help maintain a healthy mental landscape.

Resilience in the face of health challenges doesn't come from ignoring the difficulties, but rather from acknowledging them and affirming your ability to cope and thrive. Surround yourself with supportive peers, seek counseling if needed, and remember, vulnerability is not a weakness.

Personalized Health

Every individual is unique, and so is their response to diabetes. Personalized medicine is gaining ground, which includes genetic testing and analysis to understand better how different bodies respond to treatments. This can help tailor medication and diet more accurately to your personal makeup, potentially increasing the efficacy of your management plan.

Planning for the Long Term

Looking ahead involves not just maintaining health but planning for the unexpected. Discuss with your family and healthcare providers about advanced care planning. Ensure that your wishes regarding healthcare are understood and respected, should you ever be unable to express them yourself.

The Community of Tomorrow

Finally, remember the strength found in community. You are not alone on this path. Local or online support groups can be invaluable as sources of shared experience and collective wisdom. Engage with these communities, share your story, and listen to others'. Together, the journey is less daunting.

Embracing the Horizon

As you continue on this path, recognize how far you have come. Each small victory, each challenge overcome, has built your resilience and knowledge. Maintaining a healthy lifestyle with diabetes after 50 is not just about managing a condition—it's about thriving, discovering, and evolving. The next steps in your health journey are yours to define.

With each new sunrise, approach your health as you do the rest of your life—with curiosity, enthusiasm, and a zest that defies any limitations. Here's to continuing your journey with confidence and joy!